The Keto Vegetarian Diet Cookbook for Beginners

The Complete Low-Carb Beginner's Guide For Vegetarians, Ketogenic Diet, Weight Loss, Reverse Disease, and Boost Brain Health.

© **Copyright 2019 - All rights reserved.**

The content contained within this book may not be reproduced, duplicated or transmitted without direct written permission from the author or the publisher.

Under no circumstances will any blame or legal responsibility be held against the publisher, or author, for any damages, reparation, or monetary loss due to the information contained within this book. Either directly or indirectly.

Legal Notice:

This book is copyright protected. This book is only for personal use. You cannot amend, distribute, sell, use, quote or paraphrase any part, or the content within this book, without the consent of the author or publisher.

Disclaimer Notice:

Please note the information contained within this document is for educational and entertainment purposes only. All effort has been executed to present accurate, up to date, and reliable, complete information. No warranties of any kind are declared or implied. Readers acknowledge that the author is not engaging in the rendering of legal, financial, medical or professional advice. The content within this book has been derived from various sources. Please consult a licensed professional before attempting any techniques outlined in this book.

By reading this document, the reader agrees that under no circumstances is the author responsible for any losses, direct or indirect, which are incurred as a result of the use of information contained within this document, including, but not limited to, — errors, omissions, or inaccuracies.

Table of Contents

Introduction

Chapter One: About The Keto Vegetarian Diet

   What Is A Keto Vegetarian Diet

   Who Should NOT Follow A Ketogenic Diet?
- Pregnant women
- Breastfeeding women
- Hypo-causing medication
- BMI

   Benefits of a Keto Vegetarian Diet
- Appetite reduction
- Weight loss
- Fat loss
- Reduces triglycerides
- Stabilises cholesterol levels
- Insulin and blood sugar levels
- Blood pressure levels

   Impact of a Keto Vegetarian Diet

Chapter Two: Food List

   What To Eat On A Keto Vegetarian Diet
- Healthy fats
- Proteins
- Carbohydrates

   Try To Avoid

   What To Drink

Chapter Three: The Keto Flu

   The Causes

   Tackle the Keto Flu
- Be patient
- Hydrate yourself

    Plenty of fatty foods
    Eat frequently
    Sufficient sleep
    Limiting carb intake

Chapter Four: The Complete Guide To Ketosis

What Is Ketosis

Ketosis Vs. Ketoacidosis

How to Get Into Ketosis

How To Know You're In Ketosis

Chapter Five: Intermittent Fasting for Beginners

What Is Intermittent Fasting?

Intermittent Fasting For Weight Loss

Intermittent Fasting Benefits

Different Popular Regimens

The 16/8 method
The warrior diet
The 5:2 diet
Eat-stop-eat protocol
Spontaneous fasting

Intermittent Fasting FAQ

Will intermittent fasting shift my body into starvation mode?
Will intermittent fasting destabilise my blood sugar levels?
What do I eat?
Are there any side effects of this diet?
How long will it take to get used to intermittent fasting?
Can I drink anything during the fasting period?
Can it be combined with any other diet?
Is intermittent fasting is safe for everyone?

Chapter Six: Keto Condiment Recipes

Zero Carb Keto Mayonnaise

Keto Pesto

Guacamole

Keto Marinara Sauce

    Alfredo Sauce
    Keto BBQ Sauce
    Sugar-Free Caramel Sauce

Chapter Seven: Ketogenic Breakfast Recipes
    Vegan Keto Porridge
    Sundried Tomato Pesto Mug Cake
    Lemon Raspberry Sweet Rolls
    Egg Porridge
    Coffee Cake
    Roasted Veggies with Fried Egg
    Coconut Flour Pancakes
    Feta & Pesto Omelet
    Keto Raspberry Ricotta Breakfast Cake
    Cream Cheese Pumpkin Pancake
    Mocha Chia Pudding

Chapter Eight: Ketogenic Beverage Recipes
    White Chocolate Peppermint Mocha
    Coconut Almond Mocha
    Vegan Bulletproof Coffee
    Bulletproof Hot Cocoa
    Blackberry Cheesecake Smoothie
    Chocolate Smoothie
    Raspberry Avocado Smoothie
    Cream and Soda Sparkler
    Green Smoothie
    Cinnamon Almond Keto Shake

Chapter Nine: Ketogenic Snack recipes

- Pesto Keto Crackers
- Broccoli Cheese Bites
- Mini Cheese Balls
- Avocado Devilled Eggs
- BBQ Roasted Almonds
- Orange Cheesecake Fat Bombs
- Neapolitan Fat Bombs
- Blackberry Coconut Fat Bombs
- Guacamole Bombs
- Savory Mediterranean Fat Bombs
- Savory Fat Bombs

Chapter Ten: Ketogenic Salad Recipes

- Tricolor Salad
- Keto "Potato" Salad
- Warm Asian Broccoli Salad
- Egg Salad
- Crispy Tofu and Bok Choy Salad
- Avocado, Almond & Blueberry Salad
- Kale and Blueberry Salad Recipe
- Ginger Asian Slaw

Chapter Eleven: Ketogenic Soup Recipes

- Classic Cream of Mushroom Soup
- Roasted Garlic Soup
- Vegetable Soup
- Paneer and Vegetable Soup

    Butternut Squash Soup

    Coconut Curry Soup

    Broccoli Cheese Soup

Chapter Twelve: Ketogenic Lunch recipes

    Collard Green Wraps

    Grilled Cheese Sandwich

    Nori Wraps

    Cheese Omelet

    Zucchini Pizza Boats

    Cheddar and Chive Soufflés

    Spiralised Carrot and Zucchini Curry Noodles

    Spiralised Daikon Miso Noodles with Tofu

    Braised Eggs with Leek and Za'atar

    Cauliflower Fried Rice

Chapter Thirteen: Ketogenic Dinner Recipes

    Vegetarian Coconut Red Curry

    Eggplant Lasagna

    Vegan Zucchini Lasagna

    Keto White Pizza

    Grilled Veggie Plate

    Zucchini "Meatballs"

    Spicy Almond Tofu

    Portabella Pizza

    Lo Mein

    Pumpkin Cheddar Risotto

Chapter Fourteen: Ketogenic Side Dish Recipes

- Zucchini Noodles with Avocado Sauce
- Broccoli and Cheese Fritters
- Keto Bread
- Creamed Spinach
- Baked Cauliflower Casserole with Goat Cheese
- Creamy Greek Zucchini Patties
- Cheesy Ranch Roasted Broccoli
- Wilted Beet Greens with Goat Cheese and Pine Nuts

Chapter Fifteen: Ketogenic Dessert Recipes
- Raspberry Lemon Popsicles
- Strawberry Popsicle
- Avocado Popsicle with Coconut & Lime
- Pumpkin pie
- Mascarpone Cheese Mousse and Berries
- Chocolate Peanut Butter Hearts
- Keto Ice Cream
- Butter Pecan Ice Cream
- No Bake Low-Carb Lemon Strawberry Cheesecake Treats
- Pumpkin Spice Crème Brulee

Chapter Sixteen: Tips To Stay Motivated

Conclusion

References

Introduction

I would like to thank you for choosing this book, "The Keto Vegetarian Diet Cookbook For Beginners: The Complete low-carb Beginners Guide For Vegetarians, Ketogenic Diet, Weight Loss, Reverse Disease and Boost Brain Health."

We all tend to lead rather hectic and stressful lives these days. Combine this with a poor diet, and it is a recipe for disaster. Health problems have become quite common, and it is primarily because of the poor diets we consume. From an increase in obesity rates to cardiovascular diseases, everything is mostly because of our unhealthy diets, which are sans nutrients. The modern lifestyle has undoubtedly made our lives more convenient, but it has also worsened our health. All the processed and convenient foods we opt for essentially wreak havoc on our body's metabolism. A sedentary lifestyle, poor nutrition, and high stress will harm our overall well being.

Well, the good news is that all this can be changed. By changing your diet and including a little exercise to your daily routine, you can turn things around. If you want to improve your overall health and meet your weight loss goals, then the answer is the ketogenic vegetarian diet. The keto diet is a high-fat and a low-carb diet. By adding and removing certain foods, you can improve your overall health. Yes, it is really as simple as that! The vegetarian keto diet will help you attain your weight loss and fitness objectives.

The keto diet offers plenty of health benefits. It can help you lose weight as well as fat, stabilize the cholesterol levels, and also regulate the blood sugar levels. A combination of these factors improves your heart health. While following a keto diet, you will notice a surge in your energy levels. So, if you want to improve your health, then this diet is a perfect choice. Apart from this, you don't have to count the calories you consume, while on the diet. The keto food choices you make will ensure that your calorie intake reduces. According to the keto diet, you must ensure that about 70-75% of your daily calorie requirement is fulfilled by fat, 20% from proteins, and the rest from carbs.

It is a popular misconception that fats are bad. Fats have been wrongly demonized, and they don't harm you. In fact, carbs and sugars are the main culprits. If you want to lose weight, then don't worry about the fats you consume and instead, start eliminating carbs. Whenever you consume carbs, they are converted into glucose by your body. However, only a portion of this glucose is readily used, and the rest is stored in the form of fat cells. If you gain weight, it is because of this mechanism. While following the keto diet, your body burns fat. The ketones produced by the liver become the primary source of energy. By starving your body of carbs, you can significantly improve your health. One of the best things about this diet is that it is sustainable in the long run, unlike a lot of other fad diets. So, not only will you lose weight, but you will be able to maintain the weight loss with ease.

By following the vegetarian keto diet, you can undoubtedly improve your overall health. All the information you might need to get started with this diet are given in this book. Not just that, all the keto vegetarian recipes included this book provides will certainly make it easier to follow the diet. The recipes given are not only simple but are quite easy to cook as well. Mainly, you will be eating your way to good health. I promise that your opinion about food and diets will change once you are done reading this book. You can improve your overall health and even lose those excess pounds you want to. However, if you want to see this improvement, you must stick to this diet for at least four weeks to form a habit.

A poor diet combined with the hectic modern lifestyles that most of us lead these days has undoubtedly compromised our health. The good news is that you can rectify this situation. By making a few simple changes to your diet, you can reap all the benefits offered by the keto diet. However, it is quintessential that you start taking corrective action immediately. The longer you take to make these changes, the more harm you do to your body. Your body has a self-repairing mechanism. By changing your diet, you can trigger this and encourage your body to cleanse itself. So, don't allow procrastination to creep in and take action immediately.

The keto vegetarian diet is the perfect solution if you want a diet that will improve your health and help you lose weight as well. It is time to act and consciously work on improving your health. In this book, you will find all the information you need about the keto vegetarian diet. You will learn about the basics of the keto diet, the keto food list, the benefits it provides, and tips to stay motivated. Apart from this, you will also find amazing recipes to ensure that you stick to this diet plan. By following the recipes given in this book, you can start whipping out healthy, delicious, and keto-friendly meals within no time. Now, all that is left for you to do is start going through the information given in this book! So, are you ready to get started? If yes, then let us get started.

Chapter One: About The Keto Vegetarian Diet

What Is A Keto Vegetarian Diet

Vegetarian diets are considered to be one of the healthiest diets. In fact, it is believed to be quite useful when it comes to weight loss. There are several new and trendy diets that keep popping up. So, if you want to expand your horizons, then the vegetarian keto diet is a good option. This diet is a variation of the traditional keto diet or the ketogenic diet. Before you learn about the vegetarian keto diet, you must understand what a conventional keto diet is all about.

Dr Russell Wilder of the Mayo Clinic is credited with the creation of the keto diet. You might not have been aware of it, but the keto diet has been around for over 80 years. It was initially used as a form of treatment for those who suffered from chronic seizures. Back in the 1920s before there was any medication for epilepsy, the keto diet was the only form of treatment available. During the 1940s, anti seizure medications were introduced, and the ketogenic diet slowly lost its popularity. However, in recent times, this diet has undoubtedly taken the world of fitness and health by a storm. A lot of people are turning toward the keto diet for their health and reducing the dependency on pharmaceutical medicines. The keto diet is essentially a high-fat and low-carb eating protocol, which enables your body to enter a state of ketosis. A high-fat diet ensures that your energy levels stay up and triggers your body's fat-burning mechanism. A wonderful thing about the keto diet is that it not only helps with weight loss, but it also helps improve your overall health.

A vegetarian diet prohibits the consumption of poultry, meat, and fish. The only two sources of animal-based foods included in a vegetarian diet are eggs and dairy products. There are various reasons why people opt for a vegetarian diet ranging from personal or religious beliefs to ethical issues. Regardless of your reasons for choosing a vegetarian diet, you can certainly improve your overall health.

The goal of the usual keto diet is to speed up the process of weight loss by enabling your body to burn fat. Traditional keto diet is high in fats and low in protein. Vegetarian diets are believed to help with weight loss, but it is quite possible for vegetarians to be overweight as well. A traditional vegetarian diet is usually heavy in carbs and deficient in fats. By filling yourself up with carbs and sugars, you will put on weight. If you want to improve your body's metabolism without depriving yourself of the food you like, then the vegetarian keto diet is a good idea. While following the vegetarian keto diet, you will mostly have to follow the rules laid down by the traditional keto diet. So, you must ensure that at least 75% of your daily calorie requirements come from fats, about 20% from proteins and the rest from carbs. By doing this, you will shift your body into ketosis, and this helps improve your overall health as well as weight loss.

It will take your body a while to get used to the vegetarian keto diet. A regular vegetarian diet is full of carbs, and the keto diet is a low-carb diet. Initially, it might be a little tricky, but it is doable. The vegetarian keto diet recipes given in this book will certainly come in handy.

Who Should NOT Follow A Ketogenic Diet?

By shifting to the ketogenic diet, you're making significant changes to your usual eating habits. You must consult with your doctor before starting the keto diet. The keto diet is pretty safe to follow. However, certain people must not attempt this diet.

Pregnant women

A baby while in the mother's womb can face certain developmental issues because of prolonged maternal ketosis. A pregnant woman's body not only has to support itself but also the baby that is developing. A diet that is restrictive like the keto diet can have a negative effect on the baby's brain development and also increase the risk of spina bifida or other neural tube defects.

If you are trying to conceive, then it is a good idea to steer clear of the keto diet. The change of a diet can be viewed as a stressor by your body. Even if you are doing this voluntarily, your body cannot differentiate between real and perceived stress. So, don't attempt a new diet if you are planning to start a family.

Breastfeeding women

The lack of studies about the safety of the keto diet on breastfeeding women makes it difficult to understand the harmful effects of ketosis and milk production. However, any drastic changes in diet are strictly forbidden when a woman is breastfeeding. Since no one knows the result of a keto diet on breastfeeding, it is better not to make any drastic dietary changes.

Hypo-causing medication

There are certain medications like insulin, glinides, and sulphonylureas, which can cause hypos. All these medicines increase the levels of insulin in your body while reducing the levels of blood sugar. Taking these medications while following the keto diet, can worsen the hypos. So, consult a doctor before you want to follow the keto diet.

BMI

If your BMI is less than 18.5, then it means that you are underweight. Until your BMI is in the healthy or normal range, be careful while following the keto diet. You can follow the keto diet to improve your overall health, but you must take precautions to avoid weight loss. Consult a dietician to come up with a healthy meal and exercise routine before you attempt any new diet.

Benefits of a Keto Vegetarian Diet

Now that you are aware of what a keto vegetarian diet is, let us look at all the benefits it provides.

Appetite reduction

A common problem that a lot of dieters face is their ongoing struggle to overcome hunger. Conquering hunger pangs ensures that you can successfully stick to any dieting protocol. The good thing about this diet is that you don't have to worry about hunger pangs since it is a high-fat and a low-carb diet. You will tend to feel full for longer than when you consume a high-carb and high-sugar diet. When you feel full, your appetite will naturally reduce. When your appetite decreases, your calorie intake also reduces.

Weight loss

During ketosis, your body burns ketones to generate energy. In ketosis, your body is essentially reaching into its fat reserves to provide energy. A regular diet rich in carbs encourages your body to burn glucose. When it starts burning fat, you will automatically lose weight. Also, your body will stay in the state of ketosis for as long as you follow the keto diet. It means your body is effectively burning fat round-the-clock. Also, when you eliminate or restrict your carb intake, it helps with weight loss. When your insulin levels reduce, your kidneys start removing excess sodium. This, in turn, means that your body starts to get rid of any excess water stored within. A combination of these factors helps you lose weight.

Fat loss

It can be quite tricky to lose fat from the abdominal region. Losing weight might be easy but burning away stored fats isn't. The keto diet facilitates weight loss as well as fat loss. All the fat stored within your body aren't the same. The health risk posed by our body fat essentially depends on its concentration as well as location. Usually, fat cells tend to accumulate under the skin and in the abdominal region. The fat present in the abdominal area is also known as visceral fat, and it's quite harmful. Visceral facts tend to restrict the movement of insulin and causes inflammation. In ketosis, your body burns fat. So, it reaches into all the reserves of fat it has stored within. Well, if you want to lose weight from your abdominal region, the keto vegetarian diet is a good idea.

Reduces triglycerides

If you want to reduce the risk of heart disease while improving your heart's health, then a health marker you must monitor is your triglyceride level. Triglycerides refer to a group of fat molecules that are present in your body. The risk of heart diseases increases as the level of triglycerides increases. The primary cause for an increase in this level is a diet high in carbs. Since a keto diet restricts or even eliminate your carb intake, you can effectively reduce the level of triglycerides in your body.

Stabilizes cholesterol levels

Cholesterol is of two types- HDL and LDL. HDL stands for high-density lipoprotein. HDL is often referred to as good cholesterol, and LDL or low-density lipoprotein is referred to as bad cholesterol. Technically, it isn't fair to call HDL cholesterol because it is alive to protein, which enables the transport of cholesterol molecules in your blood. So, there is no such thing as good or bad cholesterol per se. All the molecules of cholesterol have a similar composition. LDL and HDL enable the transport of cholesterol molecules in your body. HDL helps carry cholesterol away from your body. By consuming foods that are rich in healthy fats, you can ensure that your level of HDL increases. When the level of HDL increases, the risk of cardiovascular diseases decreases. LDL is known as bad cholesterol, and it essentially is responsible for the transportation of cholesterol molecules in your body. The higher the level of LDL, the higher the risk of cardiovascular diseases.

Insulin and blood sugar levels

Whenever you consume any carbs, your body produces insulin, which helps in converting these carbs into glucose. So, the higher your carb intake, the more insulin your body needs. The higher the level of glucose in your body; the greater the risk of high blood sugar. A high level of blood sugar is toxic for your body. However, if your body's need for insulin keeps increasing, your body starts becoming resistant toward insulin and this, in turn, can cause diabetes. By eliminating the foods which cause a surge in your blood sugar levels, you can effectively tackle diabetes.

Blood pressure levels

Hypertension is a condition where an individual's blood pressure levels are significantly high. Hypertension tends to have a negative effect on all the major organs in your body and can cause serious health problems. The keto diet helps in regulating the levels of blood pressure in your body. This, in turn, helps improve your overall health.

Impact of a Keto Vegetarian Diet

Usually, our diets are full of carbs and processed sugars. So, the primary source of energy for your body is glucose. Glucose is usually obtained from dietary carbs like sugar and starchy foods. When you consume such foods, your body breaks them down into simple sugars. Glucose has two purposes in your body — it is used to fuel your body's functions and is also stored in the liver as well as muscles in the form of glycogen.

When you limit your consumption of carbs, your body depends on an alternate source of fuel, which is readily available to it. This alternative source of fuel is fat. Your body breaks down the fat stored within to generate glucose from triglycerides and ketones are produced. While following the keto diet, your body stops depending on carbs for producing energy and instead shifts to fats. Whenever your body burns fat, it produces ketones, which are used to generate energy. Since ketones are used for producing energy, this is where the diet gets its name.

Whenever your body doesn't have sufficient glucose to produce energy, it starts burning stored fat. This process leads to the creation of ketones in the body and is known as ketosis. Ketosis is a normal and healthy metabolic process. A low-carb diet like the ketogenic diet can help trigger ketosis. Ketosis enables your body to burn any unwanted fat by forcing your body to burn through its fat stores to provide you with energy, instead of turning to carbs to do the job.

Chapter Two: Food List

What To Eat On A Keto Vegetarian Diet

Healthy fats

While following the keto diet, it is quintessential that at least 70% of your daily caloric intake comes from naturally fatty foods. Nuts and seeds are the best sources of healthy fats for a vegetarian keto diet. There are certain nuts that are high in carbs and must be avoided. So, here is a list of low-carb and high-fat nuts and seeds you can add to your diet. Macadamia nuts, walnuts, pine nuts, hazelnuts, pecans, Brazil nuts, almonds, flaxseeds, pumpkin seeds, and chia seeds. You can also add any unsweetened nut butter made from all the nuts mentioned above.

The kind of oil that you use for cooking is also essential when it comes to the keto diet. There are certain healthy oils that you must stock up in your pantry. Whenever possible, opt for cold-pressed oils since they are considered to be the healthiest and purest oils. The oils that you can opt for include avocado oil, coconut oil, olive oil, macadamia oil, flaxseed oil, and MCT oil.

There are certain non-dairy fat sources that you can include while following the vegetarian keto diet. Non-dairy fat sources include all else, cocoa butter, avocados, and coconut cream.

Proteins

About 20 to 25% of your daily caloric intake must come from proteins. There are certain animal and plant-sourced proteins that you can add to your daily diet.

However, while opting for soy products, opt for the ones which are GMO-free and are organic. Fermented soy products will make for an excellent addition to your diet. There are certain animal-sourced proteins such as dairy products (milk, yoghurt, and cheese) that can also be added to your diet. Different types of hard cheeses which are fat free you are Parmesan, Gruyere, and cheddar. Include full-fat cottage cheese and goat cheese to your diet. Apart from this, you are free to include full-fat unsweetened Greek yoghurt and regular yoghurt. Another great source of protein that you can add to your diet is eggs — they are full of nutrients, proteins, and healthy fats.

A couple of plant-based protein sources to add to your diet are tempeh, nutritional yeast, nut-based yoghurt (unsweetened), natto, and other nuts and seeds (see previous section).

Carbohydrates

When it comes to carbs, it does get a little tricky since you're following the vegetarian version of the keto diet. You need to add plenty of low-carb vegetables to your diet to ensure that your body stays in ketosis. Not just that, the low-fat wedge you add to your diet will be the source of healthy fibre. Foods that are rich in healthy fibre tend to keep you feeling full. There are certain fruits, which you can include, but you must be selective because the fructose content in fruits can take your body out of ketosis.

The vegetables that you can include are spinach, collard greens, lettuce, kale, Swiss chard, asparagus, green beans, broccoli, red cabbage, white cabbage, cucumber, bell peppers, onions, cauliflower, mushrooms, eggplant, and garlic. Apart from this, you can also include artichoke hearts, arugula, celery, bok choy, daikon radish, fennel, kohlrabi, okra, radishes, shallots, summer squash, turnips, and zucchini.

You are free to eat any sorts of berries. Berries are not only a good source of antioxidants and vitamins, but there are also low in calories. So, a couple of berries with a tablespoon of unsweetened whipped cream can make for a delicious dessert. The different berries you can include are blackberries, raspberries, blueberries, and strawberries. Apart from this, you can also consume avocados, cranberries, lemons, limes, olives, tomatoes, and coconuts.

The different sauces and condiments that you can use are chilli sauce, hot sauce, tomato ketchup, mustard, soy sauce, and vinegar. While selecting sauces and condiments, make sure that none of these contains any added sugars.

Try To Avoid

In this section, you will be given a list of foods you must avoid while following the keto vegetarian diet. You cannot consume any meat, poultry, fish, and other animal products derived from the same. The different fruits that you cannot consume are apples, bananas, plums, mangoes grapefruit, peaches, pineapples, and peaches. You must steer clear of all types of grains and starches like rice, bulgur, buckwheat, wheat, corn, barley, oats, rye, millet, sprouted grains, and amaranth.

All grains and grain-based products like cereals, pizza, pasta, bread, oatmeal, bagels, granola, crackers, muesli, and flour must be avoided. Apart from this, you must also avoid different legumes like black beans, pinto beans, navy beans, peas, chickpeas, kidney beans, and lentils. The various kinds of root vegetables you must steer clear of include sweet potatoes, potatoes, yams, parsnips, yuca, beets, turnips, and carrots.

You must avoid all sweeteners like cane sugar, maple syrup, agave nectar, aspartame, saccharine, corn syrup, and Splenda. Any products that contain artificial sweeteners must be avoided as well. So, you must stay away from candies, chocolates, cakes, ice creams, cookies, and other desserts you can think of. Apart from this, you cannot consume any sodas, sweetened drinks, and pre-packed juices.

There are certain kinds of oils such as peanut oil, grape seed oil, canola oil, soybean oil, sunflower oil, and sesame oil that need to be avoided. Avoid all alcoholic drinks if you want to shed those extra kilos and want to become healthy. Alcohol not only contains sugars, but it also has hidden carbs in it. While opting for dairy products, keep in mind that low-fat dairy products usually have carbs or added sugars in them. So, stay away from fat-free yoghurt, skimmed cheeses, skimmed milk, and other low-fat cheeses.

What To Drink

During the initial phases of the ketogenic diet, it will take your body a while to get used to the carbohydrate restriction it will be under. Your body tends to store carbs in the form of glycogen, which in turn, retains water. Once these glycogen stores are exhausted, your body will start getting rid of the excess water weight. Apart from this, when you start removing any processed foods from your diet, it can also affect your body's electrolyte levels. If your body's electrolyte level is skewed, it will lead to severe dehydration. While following the keto diet, you must avoid all beverages that contain sugar or are sweetened with artificial sweeteners. In this section, you will learn about certain keto-friendly drinks, which you can consume daily without worrying about slipping out of ketosis.

The best drink that you can have while following the keto diet is water. In fact, regardless of whether you're following the keto diet or not, you must ensure that you drink plenty of water. On an average, your body's daily water requirement is around 8 glasses. Make sure that you carry a bottle with you at all times. Keep sipping water to ensure that your body doesn't get dehydrated. The best way to check for dehydration is by looking at the colour of your pee. If it is pale yellow or clear, then you are in the clear. However, if it is dark yellow, then it signals dehydration.

You can consume plenty of herbal teas. Herbal teas are not only low in carbs, but they also don't have any calories. That is, provided you don't add any sugar or other sweeteners to it. Green tea is rich in antioxidants and improves your body's ability to burn fat. There are several herbal teas like chamomile tea or peppermint tea, which help in reducing your stress levels as well. Have a cup of chamomile tea before going to bed to improve the quality of sleep.

If you are getting bored with drinking water, then you are always free to have seltzer or sparkling water. However, you must avoid tonic water. Adding a little bit of lemon juice or even slices of lemon can spruce up a boring glass of sparkling water.

If you like drinking coffee and cannot do without your morning cup of coffee, then don't worry. You're free to drink coffee as long as you don't add any sugar or artificial sweeteners to it. You can, however, use unsweetened heavy cream if you want. The best idea is to drink black coffee. Keep an eye on your caffeine intake. Coffee tends to have a diuretic effect on your body, and too much caffeine will deprive your body of the essential electrolytes. So, keep drinking water if you're consuming a lot of coffee.

You can also add different types of nut milk to your coffee.. The best options available are almond milk, cashew milk, and coconut milk. One cup of any nut milk contains only about one gram of carbs. So, you can start supplementing regular milk with nut milk.

A steaming cup of vegetable broth is not only filling, but it is keto-friendly as well. In fact, you can cook up some vegetable broth and added sauces, soups, or any other curries at home.

The list of items given in this section will help ensure that your body stays thoroughly hydrated.

Chapter Three: The Keto Flu

The Causes

There are different benefits that the keto vegetarian diet offers. However, it will certainly take a while for your body to get accustomed to the new diet. The only major side effect of the keto diet you must watch out for is the keto flu. It is also known as the induction flu. The keto flu goes away as soon as your body gets used to the keto diet.

The common symptoms of the keto flu include mild headaches, lethargy, nausea, tiredness, and an inability to concentrate for prolonged periods. Apart from this, you might also experience mild insomnia, constipation, mild cramps, and bad breath. You may or may not experience one or more of these symptoms. Even if you do, you can easily tackle these symptoms. Before learning about tips to tackle the keto flu, it is important that you understand the causes of the keto flu.

A diet that is high in processed foods and carbs can be rather addictive for your body. So, shifting to the keto vegetarian diet can be a significant change for your body. Your body usually uses glucose to provide energy. When you change your diet to the keto diet, your body needs to get used to burning fat instead of glucose for providing energy. It isn't an easy change for your body. So, be patient with yourself and give yourself the necessary time you need to get accustomed to this dietary change. The keto diet tends to have a diuretic effect on your body, which means your body essentially starts getting rid of any excess water along with sodium which is stored within. When this happens, it can cause constipation as well as mild cramps. Ketones tend to cause bad breath. However, this goes away as soon as your body gets used to ketosis.

Tackle the Keto Flu

The keto flu is quite real. However, the good news is that you can easily tackle it by following the tips given in this section.

Be patient

It can take your body anywhere between one week to 10 days to get used to the keto diet. As your body starts to acclimatised to this diet, any symptoms of the keto flu will also go away. So, be patient with your body. Remember that your body has been conditioned to a certain diet, and now you have completely changed. Every change requires some time for adjustment, and it's applicable to your body too.

Hydrate yourself

Since the keto diet has a diuretic effect on your body, it is quintessential that you keep yourself thoroughly hydrated. As a rule of thumb, consume about eight glasses of water daily. This also ensures that you don't overeat. By hydrating your body, you can easily get rid of some of the symptoms of the keto flu and improve your overall health. Also, your body will rid itself of any sodium stored within. So, make it a point to replace all the lost salts from your body. You can add electrolytes to the water you consume. If you start craving for salty foods, then it's a signal that your body needs some sodium. Your body knows what it needs, listen to it!

Plenty of fatty foods

While following the keto diet, you need to ensure that at least 70% of your caloric intake comes from naturally fatty foods. If you limit your intake of fatty foods, you will shift your body into starvation mode. Don't do this. Limit your intake of carbs but don't avoid naturally fatty foods. If you don't provide your body with the necessary calories it needs, it will shift into starvation mode. Once this happens, not only will your body stop burning fat, but it will also start storing fat.

Eat frequently

Don't worry that you have to restrict yourself to just three meals per day. Eat as much as you want but ensure that you only eat until you are full. Don't overeat. You can have small and regular meals if you want. By doing this, you are giving your body a constant supply of energy; however, make sure that the foods you consume are keto-friendly.

Sufficient sleep

The lack of proper sleep can also make you feel tired and lethargic. It can also bring on mild headaches. You might experience mild insomnia during the initial phases of the diet. If you ensure that you reduce your stress levels and tire yourself out physically, then you can get good quality sleep. Make it a point that you sleep for at least eight hours every night. Once your body gets used to the keto diet, you don't have to worry about all of this.

Limiting carb intake

You must be mindful of your carb intake, especially if you want your body to enter ketosis. If you consume too many carbs, your body will never get used to ketosis. The best way to overcome the keto flu is to speed up the process of induction of ketosis. By following the tips given in this section, you can ensure that you don't experience or at least limit the side effects of the keto diet.

Chapter Four: The Complete Guide To Ketosis

What Is Ketosis

Usually, your body is used to using glucose or sugar for generating energy. However, most of the cells in your body can also function while using other sources of fuel. While following a low-carb diet, your body starts using fatty acids instead of glucose for providing energy. When your carb intake is low, your internal reserves of glycogen depletes, and there is a decline in the production of insulin. This, in turn, allows your body to start burning fat to generate energy. Your liver converts a portion of these fats into ketones. The three ketones produced by the liver are acetone, acetoacetate, and BHB (beta-hydroxybutyrate). The level of carb restriction you must follow for inducing ketosis differs from one individual to another. Some people might need to make sure that the net carb intake is restricted to less than 20 grams per day, while others can attain ketosis by consuming more carbs.

Ketosis is a nutritional process that is characterised by a concentration of ketone bodies in your blood. Stable levels of insulin and blood glucose often accompany it. Acetoacetate and BHB are the primary ketone bodies that are used for providing energy. As mentioned, ketosis occurs when your body starts metabolising fatty acids or ethanol when there is an absence of glucose. Ketosis is the opposite of glycolysis. In glycolysis, your body starts storing fact because of the high levels of insulin. When the levels of insulin are high, it essentially blocks the release of any fat from the adipose tissues. While in ketosis, your body has easy access to these fat reserves. Ketosis is merely your body's psychological adaptation to the low-carb diet like the keto diet.

It will take your body a while to get into ketosis. While your body gets acclimatised to ketosis, you might experience certain side effects. Most of these side effects are temporary and will go away as soon as your body gets used to the keto diet. The side effects of ketosis are the same as the side effects of the ketogenic diet. So, for more information about this topic, refer to the previous chapter about the keto flu.

Ketosis Vs. Ketoacidosis

Ketosis and ketoacidosis might sound the same, but they aren't. Diabetic ketoacidosis or DKA is a complication related to type-1 diabetes. When the levels of ketones, as well as blood sugar, are dangerously high, it can cause a potentially fatal condition referred to as ketoacidosis. The combination of ketones and blood sugar makes your blood turn acidic, which in turn, has a negative effect on your liver as well as kidneys.

DKA can develop in less than 24 hours. It is quite common in those who have type 1 diabetes and whose bodies to produce any insulin whatsoever. There are several things, which can cause DKA like an improper diet, inadequate dose of insulin or even any illness. On the other hand, ketosis merely refers to a metabolic state where your body burns ketones for providing energy. Ketosis is not harmful. By following a low-carb diet or even by fasting, your body can enter ketosis with ease. Ketosis is defined by higher than usual levels of ketones in your blood or urine. However, the level of ketones is not high enough to cause ketoacidosis. When your body starts to burn the internal reserves of fact, it produces ketones.

The common symptoms of ketosis include bad breath, mild headaches, and tiredness. The symptoms of ketoacidosis are quite extreme. If you have ketoacidosis, you might experience extreme thirst, nausea, stomach pains, tiredness, bad breath, shortness of breath, dehydration, frequent urination, and even feelings of confusion. The symptoms of ketoacidosis can also be the first sign that you might be suffering from diabetes.

A low-carb diet of intermittent fasting can help trigger ketosis. However, improper management of diabetes is the main trigger for ketoacidosis. For instance, if someone with diabetes misses more than one dose of insulin or doesn't take the right amount of insulin, it can lead to ketoacidosis. Ketoacidosis can also be caused because of severe dehydration, acute illnesses, some medication, misuse of drugs, malnutrition, excessive consumption of alcohol, or even stress.

If the level of ketones in your blood at less than 0.6mmol/l, then it suggests normal to low level of ketosis. When the level of ketones goes above this range, then actual ketosis has set in. If the level of ketones is between 0.6 to 1.5mmol/l, your body is in a moderate state of ketosis. If the level of ketones is between 1.5 to 3.0 mmol/l, then it suggests that you are at a high risk of developing DKA. You must immediately seek medical help if the level of ketones is more than 3.0 mmol/l.

How to Get Into Ketosis

Ketosis is a helpful metabolic process, and it is quite natural. Do you want to learn about ways in which you can trigger ketosis? If yes, then read on!

The first step to enter ketosis is following a low-carb or no-carb diet. By following a low-carb diet like the keto, you can make sure that your body starts burning fat.

The consumption of coconut oil can also enable your body to enter ketosis. Coconut oil contains MCTs or medium-chain triglycerides. Unlike usual facts, MCTs are quickly absorbed by the body and are taken directly to the liver. Once MCTs reach the liver, they are rapidly converted into ketones for providing energy. You can start with something as simple as one teaspoon of coconut oil per day and then slowly make your way to maybe two or three tablespoons per day.

Exercising is good for weight loss as well as for improving your overall health. Apart from this, increasing your physical exercise can also help trigger ketosis. So, amp up your physical activity for entering ketosis. Whenever you're exercising, you force your body to exhaust its internal reserves of glycogen. Once the glycogen stores are empty, your body will start burning fat to create energy. If your carb intake is minimised, then your liver will increase its production of ketones, which helps trigger ketosis.

Fats have been wrongly demonised. A low-carb and high-fat diet like the ketogenic diet, can increase your levels of ketones. So, make it a point to consume plenty of healthy fats to improve the levels of ketones in your body.

Fasting for short periods can also help trigger ketosis. Whenever you tend to fast for prolonged periods, your body starts utilizing its glycogen reserves. Once it's out of these reserves and you don't consume any food, your body will start burning fat, which will trigger ketosis. So, following any of the protocols of intermittent fasting is a good idea. Intermittent fasting is a dieting protocol, which alternates between periods of eating and fasting. You will learn more about intermittent fasting in the subsequent chapters.

If you want to attain ketosis, you must ensure that you are consuming sufficient protein. However, consuming too much protein will do your body no good. Your protein intake must be such that it helps maintain your muscle mass without kicking your body out of ketosis.

How To Know You're In Ketosis

There are different ways in which you can check whether ketosis has set in or not. You can check the level of ketones in your blood, use a breath acetone meter or even use urine test strips.

Measuring the level of ketones in your blood provides the most accurate readings. Usually, it involves a finger prick test when a drop of your blood is placed onto a test strip, which is then inserted into the keto meter. After a couple of seconds, the device provides the number of ketones in your body. The only disadvantage of using this method is that it always requires a finger prick for obtaining the reading. The device used to measure ketones in the blood costs about $30, and each test strip can cost anywhere between $1-$3.

Testing your urine for ketones is also a good idea. This method is not expensive and is non-invasive. Apart from this, you can easily obtain a urine ketone test kit from any pharmacy. However, the results provided by this test are accurate. After a while, as your body gets used to this diet, the level of ketones in the urine will reduce.

The third option available is to test your breath for ketones. To do this, you will need a handheld device like the Ketonix. The breath keto meters measure the level of acetone present in your breath and provide the readings about the level of ketosis. However, the results produced by these devices aren't that accurate. Also, purchasing a breath keto meter is a one-time investment.

If you want to test your level of ketosis, then opting for a blood test is the best way to go.

Chapter Five: Intermittent Fasting for Beginners

What Is Intermittent Fasting?

Intermittent fasting is a dieting protocol that alternates between periods of fasting and eating. The concept of fasting is not foreign and has been around since prehistoric times. Most of us tend to fast on a daily basis and might not even realize it. For instance, your body is effectively on a fast while you are sleeping. While following intermittent fasting, you merely need to extend this duration of the fast. If you don't like eating breakfast and usually have your first meal at noon, and your last one at 8 pm, then you are effectively fasting for around 16 hours a day. This is one of the most popular methods of intermittent fasting. Unlike several other dieting protocols, intermittent fasting doesn't place any dietary restrictions. This diet concentrates mostly on *when* you eat, and not *what* you eat. One of the major benefits of intermittent fasting is that it is quite flexible. It can easily be combined with any other dieting protocol. One of the simplest ways to enable your body to enter ketosis is by following intermittent fasting. If you want, you can combine the keto diet with intermittent fasting. Once you learn about the different types of intermittent fasting protocols, you must select one of the methods. Once you select a method, you must ensure that the food you eat during the eating window is keto-friendly. If you want to improve your overall health and speed up the process of ketosis, then intermittent fasting is a great idea.

Intermittent Fasting For Weight Loss

Intermittent fasting has become a rather popular method for weight loss in the recent past. You essentially need to fast for short periods while following intermittent fasting. When you fast for short periods, you tend to consume fewer calories than useful. This, in turn, helps you lose weight. You can select any of the methods of intermittent fasting according to your needs. You will continue to lose weight while following this protocol, provided you don't make any attempts to compensate for the fasting period by bingeing on unhealthy junk during the eating window.

Before you start learning about intermittent fasting, it is quintessential that you understand the difference between the fasted and fed state. Most of us are used to snacking constantly. When you keep eating, your body is in a fed state. In this state, your body produces insulin and encourages the storage of calories in the form of fat. When there is insulin in your bloodstream, your body doesn't burn any fat. If you keep eating, your body is essentially in this state throughout the day. When you don't snack between meals, you are encouraging your body to reach into its internal reserves of fats to provide energy. In a fasted state, your insulin levels are quite low, and this, in turn, encourages your body to start burning fat cells to provide energy. Only when your body is in a fasted state will you be able to reap all the benefits offered by intermittent fasting. It can take anywhere between eight to 12 hours per your body to enter a fasted state. So, intermittent fasting is a good idea.

Your body tends to store some energy or calories in the form of fat cells. When you don't eat anything for a while, there are several changes that take place in your body. Most of these changes are related to your body's metabolism. When you're fasting, your level of insulin decreases. When your insulin level is low, your body burns any accumulated fat present within. While you are fasting, your body also starts releasing human growth hormone or HGH. HGH enables your body to start burning fat while retaining lean muscle. When you fast for short durations, your body's metabolism gets a good boost. Apart from this, intermittent fasting helps reduce your calorie intake, which will help you lose weight. If you don't try to compensate for the fasting period by overeating during the eating period, you will be fine. For instance, if you're used to consuming about 3000 calories spread over six meals, then your calorie intake will naturally reduce when you consume only three meals. When your calorie intake decreases and your calorie expenditure increases, your body stays in a calorie deficit. A calorie deficit is quintessential for losing weight. One of the good things about intermittent fasting is that it is not only helpful for losing weight, but it also enables maintenance of the weight loss.

Intermittent Fasting Benefits

Intermittent fasting is a brilliant diet, and, in this section, you will learn about the ways in which intermittent fasting can improve your health.

One of the main benefits of intermittent fasting is that it is a very flexible diet. There are various protocols of intermittent fasting and you are free to select any method that appeals to you. This isn't a restrictive diet, and you can select one according to your convenience. You don't have to worry about foregoing your social life while following any of the methods of intermittent fasting. Also, this diet is customisable. For instance, while following the 16/8 protocol, you must ensure that you fast for 16 hours per day. You are free to decide when and how you want to fast. Since this diet doesn't provide any dietary restrictions, you are free to eat whatever you want, provided you make healthy food choices.

Type II diabetes has become another common health problem these days. In this condition, your blood sugar levels are quite high, and your body starts becoming resistant to insulin. Anything that helps reduce the resistance to insulin can help in regulating the levels of blood sugar in your body. Intermittent fasting can help reduce your body's insulin resistance. So, by following this diet, you can effectively manage type II diabetes.

When you fast for short durations as specified by intermittent fasting, there are different cellular changes that take place in your body. One of the most beneficial changes is that it triggers autophagy. Autophagy is a natural process wherein your body clears and cleanses itself from within. During autophagy, your body rids itself of any damaged cells, proteins, and toxins from within. When this happens, it creates space for new and healthy cells. Apart from this, autophagy also helps in improving your immunity.

A lot of people opt for intermittent fasting because of the weight loss benefits it offers. When your calorie intake decreases, you will lose weight. A calorie deficit is a condition wherein your calorie expenditure is more than your calorie intake. When you skip a couple of meals, your calorie intake will naturally decrease. You don't have to count the calories you consume while following this diet. Calorie reduction is one of the consequences of intermittent fasting.

Oxidative stress is one of the primary causes of inflammation. Oxidative stress occurs when any unstable molecules present in your body react with helpful proteins or DNA molecules and damage them in the process. Intermittent fasting improves your body's resistance to oxidative stress. This helps reduce inflammation. Inflammation is helpful up to a certain extent. Chronic inflammation is a painful condition which can worsen your overall health.

The rate of heart disease has been steadily increasing. Most of the health markers are associated with an increase or decrease in the risk associated with heart diseases. Intermittent fasting helps improve various risk factors like blood pressure, level of triglycerides, good cholesterol, and also helps stabilise the levels of blood sugar. A combination of all these factors helps improve your heart's health.

Different Popular Regimens

There are different methods of intermittent fasting and the most popular ones are discussed in this section.

The 16/8 method

One of the most popular forms of intermittent fasting is the 16/8 method. As mentioned earlier, you are effectively fasting while asleep. The 16/8 method is an extension of this fasting period. While following this method, you are required to fast for 16 hours a day. So, the eating window is restricted to just about eight hours. In these eight hours, you can easily consume three healthy and wholesome meals. This is perhaps one of the simplest protocols of intermittent fasting. It is especially convenient if you are habituated to skipping breakfast daily. If you skip breakfast and have the first meal at noon and the last one at 8 in the night, you will be fasting for 16 hours. You are free to schedule your day according to your convenience as long as you fast for 16 hours. If you like to wake up early in the morning and exercise, then maybe you can have breakfast at around 10 am and your last meal at 6 pm. Once the eating window ends, you must not consume any solid food until the fasting window ends. However, during the fasting period, you are free to consume plenty of calorie-free beverages. You can drink water, black coffee, and herbal teas. As long as you don't consume any calories, it is good. The idea is to enable your body to stay in a fasted state for prolonged periods. When you consume calories, your body will shift into a fed state.

The warrior diet

If you like the idea of snacking all day long, then this diet might appeal to you. By following the warrior diet, you are free to consume small quantities of raw fruits as well as vegetables throughout the day. At night, you need to eat one single hearty meal. If you want, you can fast throughout the day and feast at night. The feeding window in this diet extends for only about four hours. While following this protocol of fasting, the food choices you make must be quite similar to the ones you would make while following the paleo diet. Essentially, it means that you can eat everything that was accessible to our caveman ancestors back in the palaeolithic era. While following the warrior diet protocol, you are required to consume whole and unprocessed foods. If something looks like it was produced in a factory, then you must avoid it. You will be following a high-fat and low-carb diet, just like the keto diet. If you opt for this method of intermittent fasting, then you cannot consume any sugars, carbs, or processed foods.

The 5:2 diet

If you don't like the idea of having to fast daily, then the 5:2 diet will appeal to you. While following this protocol, you must make sure that you eat like you normally would five days a week and fast on the other two days. On these two days, you must ensure that your calorie intake doesn't exceed 500 calories. You're free to consume 500 calories in the form of a single meal obviously or light meals spread across the day. If you are uncomfortable with the idea of fasting all day long or fasting daily, then this is the perfect fit for you. You are free to decide the days of the fast. Keep in mind that you are not allowed to fast on two consecutive days. For instance, if you fast on Monday, then don't fast until Wednesday or Thursday. This diet will help you lose weight and attain all the other benefits offered by intermittent fasting, provided you don't binge on unhealthy foods on the non-fasting days.

Eat-stop-eat protocol

According to the eat-stop-eat protocol of intermittent fasting, the period of fasting extends to 24 hours at a stretch. You can fast either once or twice a week. However, while scheduling the days of the fast, ensure that they are not on consecutive days. For instance, if you start your fast after dinner on Tuesday night, then you are required to fast until dinner on Wednesday night. You can plan your days as you want. The only condition is that you are required to fast for 24 hours at a stretch. You cannot consume any food during the fasting period, which will shift your body into a fed state. If you feel like it, you can certainly consume all sorts of calorie-free drinks during the fasting window. If you want to lose weight by following this method of intermittent fasting, then you must ensure that you eat healthy and wholesome foods during the feeding window. The only problem with this method of fasting is that it might be a little tricky for anyone who has never observed a fast before. If you want to follow this protocol, then it is a good idea to start with one of the simpler forms of intermittent fasting like the 5:2 diet or the 16/8 protocol. Once you are comfortable with either of those methods, you can progress to the eat-stop-eat protocol. While following this method of intermittent fasting, make sure that your fasting period doesn't go beyond 48 hours and that you don't fast on two consecutive days.

Spontaneous fasting

As is obvious from the name, you are required to fast spontaneously. There will be times when you don't feel like eating a meal because you are not hungry or are preoccupied with some work. At such times, just skip a meal. Only eat whenever you are hungry. Start listening to your body and eat when you're hungry, and only eat until you are full. Spontaneous fasting is quite simple. There are no hard and fast rules about fasting. It is merely about skipping a meal whenever you feel like. You will not do yourself any harm by foregoing a couple of meals; however, you must ensure that the other meals you consume during the week are all healthy and wholesome. If you skip meals and don't provide your body with sufficient nutrition, you will only harm your health.

Intermittent Fasting FAQ

In this section, we will be addressing common FAQs about intermittent fasting.

Will intermittent fasting shift my body into starvation mode?

Your body will not burn any fat if you keep eating after every couple of hours from the time you wake up until the time you go to sleep. If you keep consuming food, then your body will merely burn the food that you eat and store the rest. Whenever you are fasting, your body burns fat to provide energy. So, even when you're not eating, your body is essentially burning fat. So, you don't have to worry about your body entering starvation mode.

Will intermittent fasting destabilise my blood sugar levels?

Unless you suffer from hypoglycemia, you don't have to worry about any fluctuations in your blood sugar levels. If you're feeling weak and dizzy, then feel free to eat something immediately. If you skip your breakfast or maybe one meal a day, it will not harm your blood sugar levels. Your blood sugar levels will stay stable when your body starts burning fat.

What do I eat?

Intermittent fasting doesn't provide any dietary restrictions per se. However, this doesn't mean that you are free to eat whatever you want. If you binge on all sorts of unhealthy foods during the eating window, you will never be able to reap any of the benefits offered by intermittent fasting. During the eating window, ensure you consume foods that are healthy and wholesome. Try to limit your carb intake and increase the intake of healthy fats as well as protein-rich foods. You must plan your meals such that your tummy stays full during the fasting period. So, you must start making conscious decisions about the kind of food you eat and avoid. For instance, if you eat a bag of chips, you will feel hungry within no time. However, if you eat a bowl of salad that is well rounded with protein and fibre sources, you will feel fuller for longer. So, it is all about making healthy food choices.

Are there any side effects of this diet?

There aren't any major side affects you must be worried about by following intermittent fasting. Your body will need some time to get used to any new diet you wish to follow. While it is transitioning to the new diet, you might experience mild headaches or even feel a little lightheaded. However, all of this will go away once you get used to intermittent fasting. If you want to avoid these side effects, then make sure that you keep your body hydrated. Another tip which will come in handy is that you must start listening to what your body wants. If you ever feel hungry before the fast ends, it is okay to break the fast early. Don't start beating yourself up about it.

How long will it take to get used to intermittent fasting?

Your body can take anywhere between one week to 10 days to get used to intermittent fasting. The time taken will vary from one individual to another. Also, this period tends to differ based on your metabolism and your usual diet. While your body acclimatises to this diet, ensure that your exercising schedule isn't too stressful. A change in diet is a major overhaul for your body. Indulging in excessive exercising will only increase the stress on your body. A combination of these factors will do you more harm than good.

Can I drink anything during the fasting period?

While fasting, the one thing you must remember is that you cannot consume any calories. So, as long as you consume any calorie-free beverages, you are good to go. You can drink plenty of water, black coffee, and herbal teas. In fact, try to include at least a cup of green tea to your daily diet. Green tea is not only full of antioxidants, but it also encourages your body to start burning fat. Anything that doesn't have calories is permissible.

Can it be combined with any other diet?

The great thing about intermittent fasting is the flexibility it offers. Since there are no dietary restrictions it provides, you can easily combine it with any other dieting protocol like the vegetarian keto diet. Select a protocol of intermittent fasting and during the eating window, the food you must consume will be according to the food list discussed in the previous chapter.

Is intermittent fasting is safe for everyone?

A healthy adult can opt for intermittent fasting. However, there are some people who must not attempt intermittent fasting. Women who are trying to conceive, are pregnant or breastfeeding must not attempt any protocol of intermittent fasting. In fact, it is a good idea not to make any drastic dietary changes or follow any restrictive patterns of eating. If you have any pre-existing health or medical issues related to your kidney or liver, then don't attempt fasting. Also, if you are dependent on any medication, suffer from bouts of weakness, are malnourished, have high blood pressure or any other health conditions, consult your doctor before you attempt fasting. Apart from this, if you have had any history of eating disorders or are recovering from an eating disorder, then don't fast until you have made a full recovery.

Chapter Six: Keto Condiment Recipes

Zero Carb Keto Mayonnaise

Makes: About 2 cups/475 ml

Nutritional values per serving: 1 tablespoon

Calories – 95, Fat – 11 g, Total Carbohydrates – 0 g, Net Carbohydrates – 0g, Protein – 0 g

Ingredients:

- 6 tablespoons apple cider vinegar
- 2 egg yolks, at room temperature
- 2 tablespoons lemon juice
- ½ teaspoon garlic powder
- 1 ½ cups avocado oil
- ½ teaspoon salt or to taste
- ½ teaspoon paprika

Method:

1. Add all the ingredients except oil into a blender and blend until creamy and smooth.

2. With the blender motor running, pour the oil in a thin drizzle, through the feeder tube of the blender jar. Blend until the oil emulsifies.

3. Pour into a glass jar. Secure the lid and refrigerate until further use, this will last for 4-5 days.

Keto Pesto

Makes: About ¾ cup/180 ml

Nutritional values per serving: 1 tablespoon

Calories – 79, Fat – 8.09 g, Total Carbohydrates – 0.84 g, Net Carbohydrates – 0.73 g, Protein – 1.22 g

Ingredients:

- ¾ cup/180 ml fresh basil
- 6 tablespoons parmesan cheese, grated
- ½ teaspoon garlic, minced
- 1/3 cup/80 ml olive oil
- 1 teaspoon tomato paste
- 3 tablespoons pine nuts, toasted
- Salt and pepper, to taste

Method:

1. Toss the basil, cheese, garlic, tomato paste, pine nuts, and salt and pepper into a blender and blend until smooth.

2. With the blender motor running, pour the oil in a thin stream through the feeder tube of the blender jar. Blend until well incorporated.

3. Transfer into a glass jar. Fasten the lid. Refrigerate until use. It can last for 2 days.

Guacamole

Makes: About 1 cup/240 ml

Nutritional values per serving: 1 tablespoon

Calories – 16.56, Fat – 1.41 g, Total Carbohydrates – 1.11 g, Net Carbohydrates – 0.48 g, Protein – 0.23 g

Ingredients:

- 1 whole Hass avocados, peeled, de-seeded, mashed with a fork
- 1 small jalapeno pepper, finely sliced
- ½ tablespoon lime juice or to taste
- ½ cup/120 ml finely chopped fresh cilantro
- 1 tablespoon pre-made salsa
- 1 small red onion, finely chopped
- ½ teaspoon sea salt
- Black pepper to taste

Method:

1. Toss all the ingredients in a bowl. Season as per taste, add lemon juice if required.

2. Cover and chill for a while for the flavors to blend in. It can last for 2-3 days.

Keto Marinara Sauce

Makes: About 3 cups/710 ml

Nutritional values per serving: 1 tablespoon

Calories – 27, Fat – 2 g, Total Carbohydrates – 2 g, Net Carbohydrates – 1 g, Protein – 0 g

Ingredients:

- 4 tablespoons olive oil
- 4 teaspoons onion flakes
- 4 teaspoons finely chopped oregano
- 4 teaspoons erythritol
- 2 teaspoons salt
- 2 teaspoons pepper
- 2 tablespoons red wine vinegar
- 2 cloves garlic, sliced

- 4 teaspoons finely chopped thyme
- 1.36 kg / 48 ounces tomato puree
- ¼ cup finely chopped vinegar

Method:

1. Heat a saucepan over medium flame. Add oil and once it heats, add the garlic and sauté it until it starts becoming brown.
2. Add onion flakes, oregano and thyme and stir for a couple of minutes.
3. Stir in the puree, erythritol, salt, pepper and vinegar. Let it simmer for 5-6 minutes.
4. Remove from heat. Add parsley and stir. Cool completely.
5. Transfer into a glass jar. Fasten the lid. Refrigerate until use. It can last for 3-4 days.

Alfredo Sauce

Makes: About 3 cups/710 ml

Nutritional values per serving: About 6 tablespoons

Calories – 410, Fat – 41 g, Total Carbohydrates – 3 g, Net Carbohydrates – NA, Protein – 9 g

Ingredients:

- 2 cups/475 ml heavy cream
- 113.4 g /4 ounces parmesan cheese , freshly grated

- 170 g /6 ounces cream cheese softened
- ½ teaspoon granulated garlic (optional)
- 4 tablespoons unsalted butter, at room temperature
- A large pinch ground nutmeg
- ½ cup/120 ml water or as required
- Freshly ground white pepper to taste
- Salt to taste
- 2 large egg yolks
- A handful fresh basil or Italian parsley, chopped (optional)

Method:

1. Add butter, garlic and cream cheese into a pot. Place the pot over low heat. Stir frequently until the mixture is well incorporated.

2. Stir in ½ cup/120 ml cream. Increase the heat to medium-low. Stir constantly until heated thoroughly.

3. Add one fourth of the parmesan cheese and mix well. Let the cheese melt.

4. Repeat steps 2-3 until all the cream and parmesan are added. Add salt, pepper and nutmeg and stir.

5. Lower the heat to low heat. Add yolk and stir constantly until the sauce thickens slightly (a couple of minutes). Turn off the heat.

6. Taste and add more seasonings if required. Add fresh herbs if using and stir.

7. Use as required or cool completely and transfer into a glass jar. Secure the lid and refrigerate it; this will last for 3-4 days.

Keto BBQ Sauce

Makes: About 4 cups/950 ml

Nutritional values per serving: 1 ½ tablespoons

Calories – 21, Fat – 1.1 g, Total Carbohydrates – 1.7 g, Net Carbohydrates – NA, Protein – 0.5g

Ingredients:

- ½ cup/120 ml Sukrin gold brown sugar substitute or any other keto-friendly sweetener of your choice
- ½ cup/120 ml white vinegar
- ½ cup/120 ml apple cider vinegar
- 1 cup/240 ml water
- 2 cans tomato paste
- 2 teaspoons onion powder
- 2 teaspoons garlic powder
- 2 teaspoons dry mustard powder
- 2 teaspoons cayenne pepper (optional)
- 4 tablespoons butter
- 2 teaspoons salt or to taste
- 2 teaspoons liquid smoke (optional)

Method:

1. Add sweetener, white vinegar, apple cider vinegar and water into a pan. Heat the pan over medium flame. Stir frequently until the mixture is well incorporated.

2. Add rest of the ingredients and mix it. Once boiled, reduce the heat to simmer and let it simmer for 20 minutes.

3. Add more water if required, to thin the sauce.

4. Taste and adjust the seasonings and vinegar if required. Turn off the heat.

5. Use as required or cool completely and transfer into a glass jar. Secure the lid and refrigerate it, this can last for 2 weeks.

Sugar-Free Caramel Sauce

Makes: 1 ½ cups/335 ml

Nutritional values per serving: 1 tablespoon

Calories – 91, Fat – 9 g, Total Carbohydrates – 0 g, Net Carbohydrates – 0 g, Protein – 0 g

Ingredients:

- ⅔ cup/160 ml salted butter
- 1 ⅓ cups/315 ml heavy cream
- 6 tablespoons Sukrin gold or any other keto-friendly sweetener of your choice
- 2 teaspoons vanilla extract

Method:

1. Add butter and sweetener into a saucepan. Place the saucepan over low flame.

2. Stir occasionally and cook until caramelized. Be careful as it can burn easily.

3. Stir in the cream and bring to a boil. Lower the heat and simmer until thick.

4. Turn off the heat. Add vanilla and whisk well.

5. Use as required or cool completely and transfer into a glass jar. Secure the lid and refrigerate it, this can last for 2 weeks.

Chapter Seven: Ketogenic Breakfast Recipes

Vegan Keto Porridge

Number of servings: 2

Nutritional values per serving: Without toppings

Calories – 249, Fat – 13.07 g, Total Carbohydrates – 19.87 g, Net Carbohydrates – 5.78 g, Protein – 17.82 g

Ingredients:

- 8 tablespoons coconut flour
- 8 tablespoons vegan vanilla protein powder
- 2-3 tablespoons erythritol or to taste
- 12 tablespoons golden flaxseed meal
- 4 cups/1 L unsweetened almond milk

To serve:

- Toppings of your choice

Method:

1. Add all the ingredients into a heavy bottomed saucepan. Place the saucepan over medium heat.

2. Stir frequently until the mixture thickens.

3. Taste and adjust the sweetener if required.

4. Divide into 4 bowls. Place the toppings on top if desired and serve.

Sundried Tomato Pesto Mug Cake

Number of servings: 2

Nutritional values per serving:

Calories – 429, Fat – 40.5 g, Total Carbohydrates – 8.22 g, Net Carbohydrates – 5.32 g, Protein – 12.34 g

Ingredients:

For the base:

- 4 large eggs
- 8 tablespoons almond flour
- 8 tablespoons butter
- 2 teaspoons baking powder

For flavoring:

1. 4 tablespoons almond flour
2. 20 teaspoons sundried tomato pesto
3. ½ teaspoon salt

Method:

1. Add all the ingredients for base and flavoring into a bowl and whisk well.
2. Divide into 4 microwave safe mugs.
3. Microwave on high for 75 seconds.
4. Remove from the microwave and cool for a couple of minutes.
5. Tap the cup lightly on your countertop to loosen the cakes. Remove from the mugs.
6. Serve with some more sundried tomato pesto if desired.

Lemon Raspberry Sweet Rolls

Number of servings: 2

Nutritional values per serving:

Calories – 272.25, Fat – 23.18 g, Total Carbohydrates – 7.52 g, Net Carbohydrates – 5.24 g, Protein – 10.04 g

Ingredients:

For lemon cream cheese filling:

- 56.7 g /2 ounces cream cheese, at room temperature
- 1 tablespoon stevia erythritol blend
- ½ teaspoon lemon extract
- ¼ teaspoon vanilla extract

- ½ teaspoon lemon juice
- 1 tablespoons butter, at room temperature
- 1 teaspoons grated lemon zest

For raspberry sauce:

- 1 tablespoon stevia erythritol blend
- ½ tablespoon water
- ¼ cup frozen raspberries
- 1/8 teaspoon xanthan gum
- 1 teaspoon lemon juice

For dough:

- ½ cup/120 ml very fine almond flour
- 1/8 teaspoon xanthan gum
- 1 small egg
- 1 cup/240 ml part-skim mozzarella cheese
- ¾ teaspoon baking powder
- ½ teaspoon vanilla extract

For lemon glaze (optional):

- 1 tablespoon butter, at room temperature
- 1/8 teaspoon vanilla extract
- ½ teaspoon lemon juice
- ¾ tablespoon unsweetened almond milk, at room temperature

- 7 g / ¼ ounce cream cheese, at room temperature
- 1 tablespoon stevia erythritol blend
- 1/8 teaspoon lemon extract

Method:

1. To make lemon cream cheese filling: Add all the ingredients for lemon cream cheese filling into a mixing bowl. Beat with an electric hand mixer until smooth and well incorporated.
2. To make raspberry sauce: Add sweetener and xanthan gum into a saucepan and whisk well.
3. Drizzle the water and lemon juice, whisking simultaneously.
4. Place the saucepan over medium-low heat. Whisking constantly, add in the frozen raspberries.
5. When the mixture begins to simmer, turn off the heat.
6. To make dough: Grease a baking dish with cooking spray or butter.
7. To create a double boiler: Place a saucepan over medium heat. Pour 2 glasses of water.
8. Place the saucepan over high heat. When water begins to boil, lower the heat.
9. Meanwhile, add almond flour, xanthan gum, stevia and baking powder into a heatproof bowl that can fit well on top of the saucepan. Whisk well.
10. Add egg and vanilla extract and whisk well. Add mozzarella cheese and whisk well. Place this bowl on top of the saucepan over the double boiler.
11. Stir constantly until the entire mixture is well incorporated and cheese melts. Turn off the heat and remove the bowl from the double boiler.

12. Place a sheet of parchment paper on your countertop. Remove the dough and place on the center of the parchment paper.

13. Place another sheet of parchment paper on the dough. Roll the dough with a rolling pin into a rectangle of about 6 x 7.5 inches. Peel off the top parchment paper.

14. Spread the lemon cream cheese filling all over the dough except ½ inch around the edges of the rectangle.

15. Spoon the raspberry sauce evenly over the lemon cream cheese filling.

16. Roll the dough starting from the longer side. Press the edges so that it is well sealed.

17. Cut the log into 4 equal pieces, crosswise.

18. Place the rolls in the prepared baking dish.

19. Bake in a preheated oven at 350° F/177° C for 24-26 minutes or until golden brown.

20. Meanwhile, make the lemon glaze as follows: Add butter and cream cheese into a bowl. Beat with an electric mixer until creamy.

21. Beat in vanilla, lemon juice, sweetener and lemon extract.

22. Add almond milk, a few drops at a time and mix well.

23. Spread the glaze on top if using and serve.

Egg Porridge

Number of servings: 2

Nutritional values per serving:

Calories – 661, Fat – 64.5 g, Total Carbohydrates – NA, Net Carbohydrates – 2.9 g, Protein – 17.3 g

Ingredients:

- 8 organic free-range eggs
- 4 packets stevia or sweetener of your choice
- Ground cinnamon to taste
- 2/3 cup/160 ml heavy cream
- 4 tablespoons butter

Method:

1. Add eggs, cream and sweetener into a bowl. Whisk well.
2. Place a nonstick pan on low heat. Add butter. When butter melts, add the beaten cream mixture.
3. Stir constantly. The mixture will begin to get thick. At one point, the mixture will begin to curdle. Immediately remove from heat.
4. Divide into 4 bowls. Sprinkle cinnamon on top and serve.

Coffee Cake

Number of servings: 2

Nutritional values per serving:

Calories – 320.75, Fat – 28.01 g, Total Carbohydrates – 6.88 g, Net Carbohydrates – 4.24 g, Protein – 12.85 g

Ingredients:

For the base:

- 3 eggs, separated
- 2 tablespoons erythritol
- 2 tablespoons whey protein powder or plant- based protein powder
- 1/8 teaspoon cream of tartar
- 85 g/3 ounces cream cheese
- 1/8 teaspoon liquid stevia
- 1 teaspoon vanilla extract

For filling:

- ¾ cup/180 ml almond flour
- 2 tablespoons butter
- 2 tablespoons erythritol
- ½ tablespoon ground cinnamon
- 2 tablespoons sugar-free maple syrup substitute

Method:

1. To make base: Add erythritol and yolks into a mixing bowl. Beat until creamy. Add protein powder, stevia, cream cheese and vanilla and whisk until well incorporated.

2. Add cream of tartar into the bowl of whites and whip until stiff peaks are formed.

3. Add half the egg white mixture into the mixing bowl and fold gently. Add the remaining whites and fold gently. Do not overbeat or else the air from the whites will dissipate.

4. To make filling: Add all the ingredients for filling into a bowl and mix until dough is formed.

5. Grease a small, round baking pan (6 inches) with cooking spray. Line with parchment paper.

6. Pour the batter into the pan. Spoon the filling over the batter. It will sink into the batter. If it does not, push it lightly.

7. Bake in a preheated oven at 325° F/165° C for 20-25 minutes or until a toothpick when inserted in the center of the cake is clean when taken out.

8. Remove the pan from the oven and cool for 15-20 minutes.

9. Cut into 4 wedges and serve.

Roasted Veggies with Fried Egg

Number of servings: 2

Nutritional values per serving:

Calories – 349, Fat – 27.3 g, Total Carbohydrates – 19.4 g, Net Carbohydrates – 11.6 g, Protein – 12.8 g

Ingredients:

For roasted vegetables:

- 8 small heads broccoli, cut into florets

- 2 large head cauliflower, cut into florets
- 1 teaspoon garlic powder
- 1 teaspoon pepper or to taste
- 2 teaspoon red pepper flakes
- Juice of 2 lemons
- 1 teaspoon salt or to taste
- 6 tablespoons extra virgin olive oil

For fried eggs:

- 4 eggs
- Salt to taste
- Cooking spray
- Paprika to taste (optional)
- Hot sauce to taste (optional)

Method:

1. To make roasted vegetables: Add cauliflower and broccoli into a large bowl. Add oil and toss. Add garlic powder salt, pepper and red pepper flakes and toss again.

2. Transfer on to a baking sheet. Sprinkle lemon juice all over the vegetables.

3. Bake in a preheated oven at 400° F/205° C for 15 minutes.

4. To make the eggs: Place a nonstick pan over medium heat. Spray with cooking spray.

5. Crack an egg in the pan and cook until the underside is done. Flip and cook the other side for 20-30 seconds. Remove the egg and place on a serving plate.

6. Repeat steps 4-5 and fry the remaining eggs.

7. Divide the vegetables and place along with the eggs. Garnish with red pepper flakes. Drizzle hot sauce (if using) and serve.

Coconut Flour Pancakes

Number of servings: 2

Nutritional values per serving:

Calories – 77, Fat – 7 g, Total Carbohydrates – 1 g, Net Carbohydrates – 1 g, Protein – 1 g

Ingredients:

- 5 teaspoons coconut flour
- 5 teaspoons unsalted butter, melted
- 5 teaspoons sour cream
- 1/8 teaspoon salt
- ¼ teaspoon vanilla extract
- Stevia drops or ½ packet stevia powder
- 5 teaspoons heavy cream
- 1 egg or 1 more if required

- ¼ teaspoon baking powder
- ¼ teaspoon ground cinnamon
- Cooking spray

Method:

1. Add butter, stevia, eggs, cream, salt and vanilla into a bowl and whisk well.
2. Add coconut flour, cinnamon and baking powder into another bowl and stir. Add into the bowl of egg mixture and mix until well incorporated. If the batter is too thick, add another egg. Let the batter rest for about 30 minutes. Your batter will be thick.
3. Place a nonstick pan over medium flame and spray some cooking spray. Pour about ¼ of batter on it. Spread the batter with the back of a spoon.
4. Cook until golden brown on both sides.
5. Repeat steps 3-4 and make the remaining pancakes.

Feta & Pesto Omelet

Number of servings: 2

Nutritional values per serving: Without serving options

Calories – 570, Fat – 46 g, Total Carbohydrates – 2.5 g, Net Carbohydrates – NA, Protein – 30 g

Ingredients:

- 4 tablespoons butter

- 4 tablespoons heavy cream
- 4 tablespoons pesto
- Pepper to taste
- Salt to taste
- 12 eggs
- 114 g /4 ounces feta cheese, crumbled
- Chopped basil to garnish

Method:

1. Add eggs and cream into a bowl. Beat well.
2. Place a skillet over medium heat. Add 1 tablespoon butter. When butter melts, pour ¼ of the egg mixture into it. Swirl the pan so that the egg mixture spreads.
3. When the omelet is nearly done, spread 1 tablespoon pesto on one half of the omelet. Scatter ¼ of the feta cheese over the pesto. Fold the other half of the omelet over the feta.
4. Cook until cheese melts and the omelet is cooked well. Carefully slide onto a plate.
5. Sprinkle some more feta on top if desired. Garnish with basil and serve with fresh, chopped tomatoes.
6. Repeat steps 2-5 to make the remaining omelets.

Keto Raspberry Ricotta Breakfast Cake

Number of servings: 2

Nutritional values per serving:

Calories – 531, Fat – 43 g, Total Carbohydrates – 14 g, Net Carbohydrates – 7 g, Protein – 18 g

Ingredients:

- 4 tablespoons coconut flour
- 8 tablespoons almond flour
- 4 eggs
- 4 tablespoons sugar-free maple syrup substitute
- 1 1/3 cups/315 ml fresh raspberries
- 8 tablespoons butter, melted
- 1 cup/240 ml ricotta cheese, softened

Method:

1. Add all the ingredients into a mixing bowl and whisk well.
2. Divide into 4 microwave safe mugs.
3. Microwave on high for 2 minutes.
4. Remove from the microwave and cool for a couple of minutes.
5. Tap the cup lightly on your countertop to loosen the cakes.

Cream Cheese Pumpkin Pancake

Number of servings: 2

Nutritional values per serving:

Calories – 656, Fat – 62 g, Total Carbohydrates – 4 g, Net Carbohydrates – 3 g, Protein – 17 g

Ingredients:

For the pumpkin butter:

- 1 tablespoon pure pumpkin puree
- 1/8 teaspoon stevia or to taste
- 6 tablespoons butter, unsalted

For the pancakes:

- 113.4 g /4 ounces cream cheese
- 4 tablespoons coconut flour
- 4 tablespoons butter
- 4 eggs
- ½ tablespoon pumpkin pie spice blend

Method:

1. To make the pumpkin butter: Place butter and pumpkin in a microwave safe dish. Mix well. Microwave on high for about 50 seconds or until well incorporated. Mix well every 10 seconds.

2. Remove bowl from the microwave. Stir in stevia.

3. To make the pancakes: Add all the ingredients for pancake into the blender. Blend until smooth. Transfer into a bowl.

4. Place a nonstick pan over medium heat. Add 1 tablespoon butter.

5. When the butter melts, pour about ¼ of the batter on the center of the pan.

6. Cook until golden brown on both sides.

7. Remove onto a plate and keep warm.

8. Repeat steps 4-6 and make the remaining 3 pancakes.

9. To serve: Place a pancake on individual serving plates. Place a little of the pumpkin butter on the pancake and serve.

Mocha Chia Pudding

Number of servings: 2

Nutritional values per serving:

Calories – 257, Fat – 20.25 g, Total Carbohydrates – 13.75 g, Net Carbohydrates – 2.25 g, Protein – 7 g

Ingredients:

- 4 tablespoons herbal coffee
- 2/3 cup/160 ml coconut cream, undiluted
- 2 tablespoons swerve sweetener
- 2/3 cup/160 ml dry chia seeds
- 4 cups/950 ml water

- 2 tablespoons vanilla extract
- 4 tablespoons cacao nibs + extra to garnish

Method:

1. Place a saucepan with water over medium heat. Add herbal coffee and simmer until the mixture boils down to half its original quantity.
2. Pour the brewed coffee through a wire mesh strainer placed over a bowl.
3. Add coconut cream, swerve sweetener, and vanilla and stir until well combined.
4. Add chia seeds and cacao nibs. Mix well.
5. Pour into 4 serving bowls. Chill for a couple of hours.
6. Garnish with cacao nibs and serve.

Chapter Eight: Ketogenic Beverage Recipes

White Chocolate Peppermint Mocha

Number of servings: 2

Nutritional values per serving:

Calories – 320, Fat – 34 g, Total Carbohydrates – NA, Net Carbohydrates – 1 g, Protein – 1 g

Ingredients:

- 680 g /24 ounces almond milk
- 2 tablespoons powdered erythritol
- 113.4 g /4 ounces cocoa butter wafers
- ¼ teaspoon peppermint extract or more to taste
- Whipped cream to top (optional)
- 4 shots espresso
- 2 teaspoons vanilla extract
- 4 tablespoons unsweetened cocoa or more to taste

Method:

1. Add almond milk in a saucepan and heat it over medium flame.

2. When the milk is steaming hot, turn off the heat. Add rest of the ingredients and whisk until cocoa butter melts and the mixture is well incorporated.

3. Divide into 4 mugs. Top with whipped cream if using and serve.

Coconut Almond Mocha

Number of servings: 2

Nutritional values per serving:

Calories – 135, Fat – 10 g, Total Carbohydrates – 5 g, Net Carbohydrates – 3 g, Protein – 4 g

Ingredients:

- 2 cups/475 ml brewed coffee
- 8 teaspoons cocoa powder
- 1 teaspoon almond extract
- 1 1/3 cups/315 ml almond milk
- 4 tablespoons coconut butter
- Stevia or erythritol to taste

Method:

1. Heat a saucepan over medium-low flame. Add all the ingredients and whisk until well combined.
2. Heat thoroughly. Divide into 4 mugs and serve.

Vegan Bulletproof Coffee

Number of servings: 2

Nutritional values per serving:

Calories – 237, Fat – 23 g, Total Carbohydrates – 7 g, Net Carbohydrates – 5 g, Protein – 3 g

Ingredients:

- 2 cups/475 ml freshly brewed hot espresso coffee
- 2 tablespoons plain almond butter, unsalted
- 2 tablespoons organic raw extra virgin coconut oil
- Stevia to taste (optional)

Method:

1. Add all the ingredients into the blender and blend until a thick froth is formed on the top.
2. Divide into 4 mugs and serve.

Bulletproof Hot Cocoa

Number of servings: 2

Nutritional values per serving:

Calories – 486, Fat – 48 g, Total Carbohydrates – 7 g, Net Carbohydrates – 3 g, Protein – 4 g

Ingredients:

- 2 cups/475 ml full-fat coconut milk
- 2 cups/475 ml filtered water
- 4 tablespoons coconut oil or MCT oil
- 8 tablespoons grass fed butter, unsalted
- 8 tablespoons raw cacao powder or cocoa powder
- 1 teaspoon ground cinnamon
- 1 teaspoon vanilla extract

Method:

1. Place a saucepan over medium heat. Add water and coconut milk and stir.
2. When it starts to boil, remove from heat and transfer into a blender. Add rest of the ingredients and blend until smooth and frothy.
3. Divide into 4 mugs and serve.

Blackberry Cheesecake Smoothie

Number of servings: 2

Nutritional values per serving:

Calories – 515, Fat – 53 g, Total Carbohydrates – 10 g, Net Carbohydrates – 6.7 g, Protein – 6.4 g

Ingredients:

- 4 cups/950 ml blackberries, fresh or frozen
- 1 cup/240 ml heavy whipping cream or coconut milk
- 4 tablespoons MCT oil or extra virgin coconut oil
- 12-16 drops stevia or to taste
- 1 cup/240 ml full-fat cream cheese or creamed coconut milk
- 2 cups/475 ml water
- 2 teaspoons sugar-free vanilla extract or ½ teaspoon pure vanilla powder

Method:

1. Add all the ingredients into a blender. Blend it until it becomes smooth.
2. Pour into tall glasses and serve with crushed ice if desired.

Chocolate Smoothie

Number of servings: 2

Nutritional values per serving:

Calories – 570, Fat – 46 g, Total Carbohydrates – 6.2 g, Net Carbohydrates – 4.4 g, Protein – 34.5 g

Ingredients:

- 8 large eggs or 4 tablespoons chia seeds or 4 tablespoons almond butter or 4 tablespoons coconut butter
- 1 cup/240 ml chocolate or plain whey protein powder or egg white protein powder
- ½ cup/120 ml heavy whipping cream or coconut milk
- 4 tablespoons MCT oil or extra virgin coconut oil
- 12-16 drops stevia extract or to taste
- 2 teaspoons ground cinnamon or vanilla extract (optional)
- 4 tablespoons cacao powder, unsweetened
- 1 cup/240 ml water
- 1 cup/240 ml ice cubes or as required

Method:

1. Add everything into a blender and blend until it turns smooth and frothy
2. Pour into tall glasses and serve cold.

Raspberry Avocado Smoothie

Number of servings: 2

Nutritional values per serving:

Calories – 227, Fat – 20 g, Total Carbohydrates – 12.8 g, Net Carbohydrates – 4 g, Protein – 2.5 g

Ingredients:

- 2 ripe avocadoes, peeled, pitted, chopped
- 6 tablespoons lemon juice
- 1 cup/240 ml frozen raspberries, unsweetened
- 2 2/3 cup/160 ml water
- 4 tablespoons swerve or any other keto-friendly sugar substitute or your choice

Method:

1. Add everything into a blender and blend until it turns smooth and frothy
2. Pour into tall glasses and serve cold.

Cream and Soda Sparkler

Number of servings: 2

Nutritional values per serving:

Calories – 206, Fat – 22 g, Total Carbohydrates – 2 g, Net Carbohydrates – NA, Protein – 1 g

Ingredients:

- 226.8 g /8 ounces heavy cream
- Sparkling flavored water, unsweetened, chilled, as required
- 7-8 tablespoons sugar-free raspberry syrup

Method:

1. Divide equally raspberry syrup and heavy cream in 4 glasses.
2. Add sparkling water, a little at a time as it will be frothy.
3. Stir and serve.

Green Smoothie

Number of servings: 2

Nutritional values per serving:

Calories – 148, Fat – 11 g, Total Carbohydrates – 13 g, Net Carbohydrates – 7 g, Protein – 2 g

Ingredients:

- 2 cups/475 ml cold water
- 1 cup/240 ml cilantro
- 1 ½ English cucumber, peeled and chopped
- 2 cups/475 ml frozen avocado

- 2 cups/475 ml baby spinach
- 2 inches ginger, peeled, sliced
- Juice of 2 lemons

Method:

1. Add everything into a blender and blend until it turns smooth and frothy
2. Pour into tall glasses and serve cold.

Cinnamon Almond Keto Shake

Number of servings: 2

Nutritional values per serving:

Calories – 255, Fat – 14 g, Total Carbohydrates – 7 g, Net Carbohydrates – NA, Protein – 29 g

Ingredients:

- 4 tablespoons almond butter
- ½ teaspoon ground cinnamon
- 4 scoops whey protein powder, unsweetened
- 4 teaspoons vanilla extract
- Ice cubes, as required
- 4 cups/950 ml almond milk, unsweetened

Method:

1. Add everything into a blender and blend until it turns smooth and frothy
2. Pour into tall glasses and serve cold.

Chapter Nine: Ketogenic Snack recipes

Pesto Keto Crackers

Number of servings: 2

Nutritional values per serving:

Calories – 210, Fat – 20 g, Total Carbohydrates – 5.5 g, Net Carbohydrates – 3 g, Protein – 5 g

Ingredients:

- ¾ cup/180 ml + 2 tablespoons almond flour
- ¼ teaspoon salt or to taste
- ½ teaspoon dried basil
- 2 small cloves garlic, pressed
- 2 tablespoons butter, chopped into small pieces
- Pepper to taste
- ¼ + 1/8 teaspoon baking powder
- 1/8 teaspoon cayenne pepper
- 1 ½ tablespoons pesto

Method:

1. Place a sheet of parchment paper over a baking sheet.
2. Add all the dry ingredients into a bowl and mix well. Add basil, pesto and garlic and mix using your hands until crumbly.
3. Add butter and mix well using your hands until dough is formed.
4. Place the dough on the baking sheet and roll the dough evenly until quite thin, like normal crackers.
5. Bake in a preheated oven at 325° F/165 ° C for 14-17 minutes or until light golden brown.
6. When done, remove from the oven and cut into 4 squares.
7. Cool completely. Store in an airtight container until use.

Broccoli Cheese Bites

Number of servings: 2

Nutritional values per serving: 3 bites

Calories – 177, Fat – 15 g, Total Carbohydrates – 3 g, Net Carbohydrates – 2.4 g, Protein – 12 g

Ingredients:

- 1 head broccoli, cut into florets
- 2 tablespoons sliced scallions
- ½ cup/120 ml grated cheddar cheese

- 1 egg
- ¼ teaspoon pepper or to taste
- Salt to taste
- ¼ cup frozen spinach, thawed, drained
- Zest of ½ lemon, grated
- 2 tablespoons grated parmesan cheese
- 3 tablespoons sour cream

Method:

1. Add broccoli into a microwave safe bowl. Sprinkle 2-3 tablespoons water.
2. Cook on High for about 3 minutes or until tender. Remove the bowl from the microwave and drain off the liquid in the bowl.
3. Set aside to cool. When cool enough to handle, finely chop the broccoli. The chopped broccoli should measure around 1 ¼ cups. Add into a bowl.
4. Add rest of the ingredients and stir until well incorporated.
5. Transfer the mixture into a square baking pan of about 8 inches that is lined with parchment paper. Spread it evenly.
6. Bake in a preheated oven at 355° F/180° C for 22-25 minutes or until light golden brown.
7. When done, remove from the oven and cut into 12 equal squares.
8. Cool completely. Store in an airtight container until use.

Mini Cheese Balls

Number of servings: 2

Nutritional values per serving: 2 balls

Calories – 94, Fat – 7.4 g, Total Carbohydrates – 2 g, Net Carbohydrates – 2 g, Protein – 5 g

Ingredients:

- 48.2 g /1.7 ounces plain almond milk cream cheese
- 48.2 /1.7 ounces goat's cheese
- 1/8 teaspoon grated lemon zest
- ½ teaspoon finely chopped fresh thyme
- 3 tablespoons roasted, chopped salted almonds

Method:

1. Place goat's cheese, cream cheese and lemon zest in a bowl.
2. Beat with an electric mixer set on medium speed until smooth. Place the bowl in the freezer for 15 minutes.
3. Add nuts and thyme into the food processor bowl and process until fine. Transfer into a bowl.
4. Divide the mixture into 8 equal portions and make balls out of it.
5. Dredge the balls in the nut mixture. Cover and chill until use.

Avocado Devilled Eggs

Number of servings: 2

Nutritional values per serving: 1 egg half

Calories – 147, Fat – 14.8 g, Total Carbohydrates – 2.5 g, Net Carbohydrates – 1.1 g, Protein – 2.2 g

Ingredients:

- 4 large eggs, hard boiled, peeled, halved lengthwise
- 3 ½ tablespoons mayonnaise
- Salt to taste
- 1 ½ tablespoons thinly sliced spring onion
- Freshly ground pepper to taste
- 80 g /2.8 ounces avocado, peeled, pitted, chopped
- 1 ½ tablespoons lemon juice or lime juice or to taste

Directions

1. Carefully scoop the yolks from the whites and add into a bowl. Set aside the whites.
2. Add avocado, lemon juice, mayonnaise, pepper and salt into the bowl of yolks and mash well with a fork.
3. Fill 2 tablespoons of this mixture in the cavities of the whites.
4. Serve.

BBQ Roasted Almonds

Number of servings: 2

Nutritional values per serving: ¼ cup

Calories – 229, Fat – 19.6 g, Total Carbohydrates – 9.3 g, Net Carbohydrates – 4.3 g, Protein – 8 g

Ingredients:

- 1 cup/240 ml almonds, soaked in water overnight, drained
- ½ tablespoon paprika
- ½ teaspoon salt or to taste
- ½ teaspoon onion powder
- ½ tablespoon olive oil
- 1 teaspoon chili powder
- ½ teaspoon ground cumin
- ½ teaspoon garlic powder
- ½ teaspoon pepper
- ½ teaspoon granulated swerve or erythritol

Method:

1. Place layers of paper towels on a plate. Spread the almonds on it. Pat the almonds dry.

2. Add the almonds into a bowl. Add rest of the ingredients and toss until well coated.

3. Place parchment paper on a baking sheet. Spread the almonds on the baking sheet.

4. Bake in a preheated oven at 300300° F/150° C for about 30-40 minutes or until dry. Stir the almonds a couple of times while it is baking. If the almonds seem wet in the center, bake for some more time.

5. Cool completely. Transfer into an airtight container until use.

Orange Cheesecake Fat Bombs

Number of servings: 2

Nutritional values per serving:

Calories – 106, Fat – 11 g, Total Carbohydrates – Trace, Net Carbohydrates – Trace, Protein – 1 g

Ingredients:

- 1 teaspoon finely grated orange zest, divided
- 1 ½ tablespoons coconut oil, softened
- 42.5 g /1.5 ounces cream cheese, at room temperature
- ¼ teaspoon lemon juice or to taste
- 10 drops liquid stevia or to taste
- 1 ½ tablespoons unsalted butter, softened

- ¼ teaspoon orange extract (optional)

Method:

1. Retain ½ teaspoon of orange zest and add rest of the ingredients into a blender and blend until smooth.

2. Transfer the mixture into 4 cupcake liners or 4 mini muffin molds. Sprinkle the retained orange zest on top.

3. Freeze until set and serve.

4. Store in the freezer until use.

Neapolitan Fat Bombs

Number of servings: 2

Nutritional values per serving:

Calories – 102, Fat – 10.9 g, Total Carbohydrates – 0.6 g, Net Carbohydrates – 0.4 g, Protein – 0.6 g

Ingredients:

- 1 ¼ tablespoons butter
- 1 ¼ tablespoons sour cream
- 1 teaspoon cocoa powder, unsweetened
- 1 ¼ tablespoons coconut oil
- 1 ¼ tablespoons cream cheese
- 1 teaspoon erythritol

- ¼ teaspoon vanilla extract
- 8 drops liquid stevia or to taste
- 1 small strawberry, finely chopped

Method:

1. Add butter, sour cream, coconut oil, cream cheese, erythritol and stevia into a bowl. Blend with an immersion blender until it becomes smooth and creamy.
2. Divide the mixture equally into 3 small bowls.
3. Add cocoa powder to the first bowl and mix well.
4. Add vanilla extract to the second bowl and mix well.
5. Mash the strawberries and add to the third bowl and mix well.
6. Pour the cocoa mixture into 4 fat bomb molds. Place the molds in the freezer for 30 minutes.
7. Remove molds from the freezer and pour the vanilla mixture over it. Place in the freezer for another 30 minutes.
8. Remove from the freezer and pour the strawberry mixture over it.
9. Freeze for a couple of hours.
10. Remove from the mold and serve immediately.

Blackberry Coconut Fat Bombs

Number of servings: 2

Nutritional values per serving:

Calories – 170, Fat – 18.7 g, Total Carbohydrates – 3 g, Net Carbohydrates – 0.7 g, Protein – 1.1 g

Ingredients:

- ¼ cup/60 ml coconut butter
- 1/8 cup/30 ml fresh or frozen blackberries or any other berries of your choice
- 5 drops vanilla extract
- ¼ cup/60 ml coconut oil
- 4-5 drops stevia or to taste
- ¾ teaspoon lemon juice or to taste

Method:

1. Add coconut oil, coconut butter and blackberries into a small pan. Place the pan over medium heat. Stir constantly until just incorporated. Turn off the heat. Cool for a few minutes.
2. Transfer into the blender. Add rest of the ingredients and blend until smooth.
3. Line a small pan with parchment paper.
4. Pour the mixture into the prepared pan.
5. Chill until firm. Cut into 4 equal squares and serve.

Guacamole Bombs

Number of servings: 2

Nutritional values per serving:

Calories – 191, Fat – 16 g, Total Carbohydrates – 8 g, Net Carbohydrates – 2 g, Protein – 5 g

Ingredients:

- 4 cookie scoops guacamole
- 1 small egg, beaten
- 1 tablespoon oil
- 6 tablespoons keto breadcrumbs

Method:

1. Place 4 cookie scoops of guacamole on a baking dish that is lined with parchment paper. Cover the dish with cling wrap and place the dish in the freezer until firm.

2. Place breadcrumbs in a bowl.

3. Place a nonstick pan over medium. Add oil and let it heat. First dip guacamole ball in egg, one at a time. Shake to drop off excess egg. Next dredge in breadcrumbs and place on the heated pan. Repeat this with the remaining guacamole balls.

4. Cook until golden brown all over. Remove from the pan and serve immediately.

Savory Mediterranean Fat Bombs

Number of servings:

Nutritional values per serving:

Calories – 164, Fat – 17.1 g, Total Carbohydrates – 2 g, Net Carbohydrates – 1.7 g, Protein – 3.7 g

Ingredients:

- 80 g /2.8 ounces cream cheese, at room temperature
- 1 ½ -2 tablespoons chopped mixture of fresh basil, oregano and thyme or 1 ¾ teaspoons dried mixed herbs
- 3 Kalamata olives, pitted, chopped
- Salt to taste
- Pepper to taste
- 1 large clove garlic, crushed
- 9.6 g / 0.32 ounce sundried tomatoes, drained
- 44 g/1.6 ounce butter or ghee, cut into small cubes, at room temperature
- 4 tablespoons grated parmesan cheese

Method:

1. Add butter and cream cheese into a bowl. Mash well.
2. Add rest of the ingredients and mix well. Refrigerate for an hour.
3. Divide the mixture into 4 equal portions and shape balls. Chill until use.

Savory Fat Bombs

Number of servings: 2

Nutritional values per serving:

Calories – 75, Fat – 7 g, Total Carbohydrates – 1 g, Net Carbohydrates – Trace, Protein – 2 g

Ingredients:

- 100 g /3.33 ounces cream cheese, at room temperature
- 4 olives, pitted, chopped
- 1 1/3 tablespoons grated parmesan cheese
- ¾ teaspoon minced garlic
- Salt to taste

Method:

1. Set aside parmesan cheese on a plate and add the remaining ingredients in a bowl and mix well. Refrigerate for an hour.
2. Divide the mix into 4 portions and shape into balls. Chill until use.

Chapter Ten: Ketogenic Salad Recipes

Tricolor Salad

Number of servings: 2

Nutritional values per serving:

Calories – 581, Fat – 50.7 g, Total Carbohydrates – 17.7 g, Net Carbohydrates – 8.6 g, Protein – 19.2 g

Ingredients:

- 600 g / 21.2 ounces medium tomatoes, sliced
- 14-16 olives, pitted, sliced
- ¼ cup pesto
- ¼ cup extra virgin olive oil
- 2 large avocadoes (400 g / 14.2 ounces), seeded, peeled, sliced
- 10 olives, sliced
- Salt and pepper, to taste
- 250 g / 8.8 ounces mozzarella, cubed
- 2 tablespoons fresh basil, chopped

Method:

1. Add all the ingredients to a large bowl. Toss well and serve.

Keto "Potato" Salad

Number of servings: 2

Nutritional values per serving:

Calories – 254, Fat – 21.1 g, Total Carbohydrates – 10.5 g, Net Carbohydrates – 7.6 g, Protein – 6.6 g

Ingredients:

For salad:

- 1 small turnip, peeled, chopped into ½ inch pieces
- 1 small celeriac, peeled, chopped into ½ inch pieces
- 1 small rutabaga, chopped into ½ inch pieces
- 1 small onion, finely chopped
- 2-3 pickled cucumber, diced
- 1 medium stalk celery, sliced
- 3 large eggs, hard boiled, peeled, chopped into bite sized pieces

Spices to boil vegetables:

- ½ tablespoon apple cider vinegar
- 1 bay leaf
- ½ teaspoons black peppercorns
- 1 teaspoon salt

For dressing:

- ½ teaspoon Dijon mustard
- 6 tablespoons mayonnaise
- 1 tablespoon pickle juice or vinegar
- ½ teaspoon celery seeds
- 1 tablespoon chives, chopped
- A handful fresh parsley, chopped
- Salt and pepper, to taste

Method:

1. Heat water over high flame in a pot. Add vinegar, peppercorns, salt, and bay leaves.
2. Add rutabaga, turnips and celeriac.
3. When it boils, lower the flame and simmer until vegetables are tender. Discard the spices and drain off the water.
4. Transfer the cooked vegetables into a bowl and let it cool completely.
5. Add rest of the ingredients of salad into the bowl of vegetables and toss well.

6. Add all the dressing ingredients in a bowl and whisk well.

7. Pour dressing over the salad. Toss well and serve.

Warm Asian Broccoli Salad

Number of servings: 2

Nutritional values per serving:

Calories – 62.63, Fat – 4.28 g, Total Carbohydrates – 4.72 g, Net Carbohydrates – 3.62 g, Protein – 1.8 g

Ingredients:

- 170 g /6 ounces broccoli slaw
- ½ tablespoon coconut aminos
- Pepper to taste
- Salt to taste
- ¼ teaspoon sesame seeds
- 1 tablespoon coconut oil
- ½ teaspoon grated fresh ginger
- ¼ cup full-fat plain goat milk yogurt
- Cilantro, chopped, to garnish

Method:

1. Place a skillet over medium high flame. Add oil; once the oil gets heated, add broccoli slaw and cover with a lid.

2. When it wilts, add coconut aminos, pepper, salt and ginger and mix well. Turn off the heat.

3. Add yogurt and stir.

4. Garnish with sesame seeds and serve.

Egg Salad

Number of servings: 2

Nutritional values per serving:

Calories – 575, Fat – 51 g, Total Carbohydrates – 7 g, Net Carbohydrates – 2 g, Protein – 20 g

Ingredients:

- 2 medium avocadoes, peeled, pitted, chopped
- 2/3 cup/160 ml mayonnaise
- 1 tablespoon lemon juice
- 1 tablespoon chopped fresh parsley (optional)
- 12 eggs, hard boiled, peeled, chopped
- 2 teaspoons Dijon mustard

- ¼ teaspoon dried dill (optional)
- Salt and pepper, to taste

Method:

1. Add the ingredients into a bowl and stir lightly.
2. Cover and refrigerate until use.
3. Serve chilled.

Crispy Tofu and Bok Choy Salad

Number of servings: 2

Nutritional values per serving:

Calories – 442, Fat – 35 g, Total Carbohydrates – 8.29 g, Net Carbohydrates – 5.7 g, Protein – 25 g

Ingredients:

For oven baked tofu:

- 20 ounces extra firm tofu, chopped into 1 inch squares
- 1 ½ tablespoons sesame oil
- 2 ½ teaspoons garlic, minced
- Juice of a lemon
- 1 ½ tablespoons soy sauce or tamari

- 1 ½ tablespoons water
- 1 ½ tablespoons red wine vinegar

For Bok Choy salad:

- 12 ounces Bok Choy, thinly sliced
- A handful fresh cilantro, chopped
- 2 ½ tablespoons soy sauce or tamari
- 1 ½ tablespoons peanut butter
- 2 small stalks green onion, chopped
- 9-10 drops stevia or to taste
- 4 tablespoons coconut oil, melted
- 4 teaspoons sambal olek
- Juice of a lime or to taste

Method:

1. To press the tofu: Place tofu over layers of paper towels. Place something heavy like a heavy bottomed pan over the tofu to drain out excess moisture. Let it remain in this position for 4-5 hours.

2. Transfer onto a cutting board and chop into square pieces.

3. Add soy sauce, sesame oil, lemon, water, garlic and vinegar into a bowl. Whisk well.

4. Add tofu into it. Mix well so that the tofu is well coated with the marinade. Place in the refrigerator for 6-7 hours.

5. Spread a parchment paper on the baking sheet. Remove the tofu from the marinade and place on the prepared baking sheet.

6. To make salad dressing: Add cilantro, soy sauce, peanut butter, green onion, stevia, coconut oil, sambal olek and lime juice into a bowl. Whisk well. Keep it aside for a while so that the flavors can set in.

7. To assemble: Place Bok Choy on a serving platter. Layer with tofu. Drizzle the dressing over it and serve.

Avocado, Almond & Blueberry Salad

Number of servings: 2

Nutritional values per serving:

Calories – 256.4, Fat – 20.2 g, Total Carbohydrates – 16.5 g, Net Carbohydrates – 7.9 g, Protein – 6.2 g

Ingredients:

- 4 cups/950 ml arugula mix
- 60 g /2.1 ounces sliced almonds
- 2 ripe avocadoes, peeled, pitted, chopped
- 4 tablespoons MCT oil (optional)
- 2 cups/475 ml Trader Joes Cruciferous crunch
- 113.4 g /4 ounces blueberries
- 7-8 tablespoons Trader Joes Green Goddess Dressing

Method:

1. Add all the ingredients into a bowl and toss well.
2. Divide into 4 plates and serve immediately.

Kale and Blueberry Salad Recipe

Number of servings: 2

Nutritional values per serving:

Calories – 191, Fat – 16 g, Total Carbohydrates – 13 g, Net Carbohydrates – 9 g, Protein – 4 g

Ingredients:

- 340 g / 12 ounces kale, roughly chopped, discard hard stems and ribs
- 2 tablespoons sliced almonds
- 2 tablespoons chopped parsley
- 4 tablespoons olive oil
- 20 blueberries
- ½ red onion, thinly sliced
- 2 tablespoons lemon juice
- Salt and pepper, as per taste

Method:

1. Add all the ingredients in a bowl and toss well.
2. Divide into 4 plates and serve immediately.

Ginger Asian Slaw

Number of servings: 2

Nutritional values per serving:

Calories – 144, Fat – 6 g, Total Carbohydrates – 19 g, Net Carbohydrates – 14 g, Protein – 4 g

Ingredients:

For coleslaw:

- 3 cups/710 ml thinly sliced red cabbage
- 3 cups/710 ml thinly sliced green cabbage or Napa cabbage
- 1 cup/240 ml shredded carrot
- 2 green onions, thinly sliced
- ½ cup/120 ml chopped cilantro

For Asian coleslaw dressing:

- ½ tablespoon olive oil
- ½ teaspoon sesame oil

- 1 tablespoon tamari
- 1 tablespoon almond butter
- 2 small cloves garlic, peeled, minced
- Zest of ½ lemon, grated
- 1-2 tablespoons lime juice
- ½ tablespoon sugar-free maple syrup
- ½ tablespoon apple cider vinegar
- ½ tablespoon rice wine vinegar
- ¾ inch fresh ginger, peeled, grated

Method:

1. Add all the ingredients for coleslaw dressing into a blender and blend until smooth.
2. Add all the vegetables into a large bowl and toss well.
3. Drizzle the dressing on top. Toss well and serve.
4. Chill and serve.

Chapter Eleven: Ketogenic Soup Recipes

Classic Cream of Mushroom Soup

Number of servings: 2

Nutritional values per serving:

Calories – 95, Fat – 4 g, Total Carbohydrates – 12.3 g, Net Carbohydrates – 7.9 g, Protein – 4.9 g

Ingredients:

- 4 cups/950 ml cauliflower florets
- 2 teaspoons onion powder
- 1 teaspoon extra virgin olive oil
- 1 medium yellow onion, chopped
- 3 cups/710 ml mushrooms, diced
- 3 1/3 cups/710 ml almond milk, unsweetened
- ½ teaspoon Himalayan pink salt
- Salt to taste
- Freshly ground pepper to taste

Method:

- Add milk, cauliflower, onion powder, salt and pepper into saucepan. Place the saucepan over medium heat.

- When it begins to boil, lower the heat and cover with a lid. Simmer until tender. Turn off the heat and blend with an immersion blender until smooth.

- Place a saucepan over high heat. Add oil. When the oil is heated, add onions and sauté until translucent.

- Add mushrooms and sauté until brown. Add pureed soup, and lower the heat and cover with a lid. Simmer for 10 minutes.

- Ladle into soup bowls and serve.

Roasted Garlic Soup

Number of servings: 2

Nutritional values per serving:

Calories –73, Fat – 2.4 g, Carbohydrates – 11.3 g, Net Carbohydrates – 9.2 g, Protein – 2.1 g

Ingredients:

- 1 large and 1 small bulb garlic

- 2 shallots, chopped

- Salt to taste

- 4 cups/950 ml vegetable broth

- 2 teaspoons extra virgin olive oil, divided
- 1 medium head cauliflower, chopped (3 1/3 cups/710 ml)
- Freshly ground pepper to taste

Method:

1. Remove the outer layers of the garlic skin and slice about ¼ inch from the top.
2. Brush with oil and place in foil. Wrap it well.
3. Roast in a preheated oven at 400° F/205° C for around 25-35 minutes. Remove from the oven and do not unwrap for a while.
4. Unwrap and squeeze the garlic so that the garlic cloves come off the skin.
5. Place a saucepan over medium heat. Add remaining oil. When the oil is heated, add shallots and sauté until light brown.
6. Add garlic cloves and rest of the ingredients and cover with a lid.
7. Lower the heat and simmer until the cauliflower is cooked.
8. Turn off the heat and cool for a while. Toss it in a blender and blend until smooth. Taste and adjust the seasoning if required.
9. Pour the soup back into the saucepan. Heat it well.
10. Serve hot in soup bowls.

Vegetable Soup

Number of servings: 2

Nutritional values per serving:

Calories – 79, Fat – 2 g, Total Carbohydrates – 11 g, Net Carbohydrates – 8 g, Protein – 2 g

Ingredients:

- 2 teaspoons olive oil
- 1 medium bell pepper, chopped
- 1 small head cauliflower, cut into 1 inch pieces
- 1 small onion, chopped
- 2 cloves garlic, minced
- 272.2 g /9.6 ounces canned diced tomatoes
- 1 teaspoon Italian seasoning
- Pepper to taste
- Salt to taste
- 2/3 cup/160 ml chopped green beans (cut into 1 inch pieces)
- 2 ½ -3 cups/710 ml vegetable broth
- 1 bay leaf (optional)

Method:

1. Heat a soup pot over medium flame and add oil. Once the oil gets heated, add onion and bell pepper and cook until onions are light brown.

2. Stir in the garlic and cook for a few seconds until aromatic.

3. Add rest of the ingredients and stir.

4. Once it boils, reduce the heat and simmer until vegetables are soft.

5. Ladle into soup bowls and serve.

Paneer and Vegetable Soup

Number of servings: 2

Nutritional values per serving:

Calories – 472, Fat – 18 g, Total Carbohydrates – NA, Net Carbohydrates – 6 g, Protein – 11 g

Ingredients:

- 4 tablespoons coconut milk
- 100 g / 3.5 ounces bottle gourd (calabash), peeled, cubed
- 4 cloves garlic, minced
- 100 g / 3.5 ounces turnip, peeled, cubed
- 200 g / 7 ounces spinach, finely chopped
- 2 teaspoons ginger paste
- ½ teaspoon ground cloves
- 1 teaspoon ground star anise

- Pepper to taste
- Salt to taste
- 8 tablespoons melted ghee
- 200 g / 7 ounces paneer or cottage cheese, chopped into small cubes
- 1 small onion, finely chopped
- 3 cups/710 ml water

Method:

1. Place a soup pot over medium heat. Add ghee. When it melts, add cottage cheese cubes and cook until brown all over.
2. Remove with a slotted spoon and set aside.
3. Add onion into the pot. Sauté until translucent. Add ginger paste and garlic and sauté until it becomes aromatic.
4. Also add star anise and cloves and mix well.
5. Add water, turnip and bottle gourd and stir. Once it starts to boil, reduce the flame and simmer until vegetables are soft.
6. Add spinach and cook for a few minutes until spinach wilts.
7. Add coconut milk, salt and pepper and cook for 5 minutes.
8. Turn off the heat. Cool for a while.
9. Transfer into a blender and blend until smooth.
10. Pour it back into the pot and heat thoroughly.
11. Ladle into 4 soup bowls. Divide paneer among the bowls and serve.

Butternut Squash Soup

Number of servings: 2

Nutritional values per serving:

Calories – 183, Fat – 12 g, Total Carbohydrates – 12 g, Net Carbohydrates – 10 g, Protein – 6 g

Ingredients:

- 1 pound butternut squash, halved lengthwise, de-seeded
- 3 cloves garlic, peeled and minced
- 1 bay leaf (optional)
- ½ teaspoon pepper or to taste
- ½ teaspoon salt or to taste
- ½ can (from a 13.5 ounces /383 g can) coconut milk
- 1 tablespoon minced fresh thyme
- 2 cups/475 ml vegetable broth
- A pinch ground nutmeg
- ¼ teaspoon ground cinnamon
- 1 tablespoon avocado oil, divided

Method:

1. Place butternut squash on a baking sheet lined with foil or parchment paper, with the cut side facing up.

2. Brush ½ tablespoon oil over it.

3. Season with salt and pepper and now turn the butternut squash, cut side facing down.

4. Roast in a preheated oven at 400° F for around 40 minutes or a knife when inserted in the pulp pierces easily.

5. Place a skillet over medium heat. Add remaining oil. When the oil gets hot, add thyme, garlic and spices and cook until it becomes aromatic.

6. Stir in coconut milk and broth. Lower the heat and simmer for about 15 minutes. Turn off the heat.

7. When the squash is cool enough to handle, scrape the pulp from the shell and add into the soup. Blend with an immersion blender until smooth.

8. Ladle into 4 soup bowls and serve.

Coconut Curry Soup

Number of servings: 2

Nutritional values per serving:

Calories – 503, Fat – 41.8 g, Total Carbohydrates – 15.8 g, Net Carbohydrates – 11 g, Protein – 25.2 g

Ingredients:

- 500 g /1.1 pounds firm tofu, cubed
- 1 inch piece ginger, peeled, minced
- 1 large red onion, chopped

- 2 medium zucchinis
- 200 g /7.05 ounces mushrooms, sliced
- 4 cups/950 ml water
- 2 large cloves garlic, peeled, minced
- 1 1/3 cups/310 ml coconut milk
- 2 vegetarian bouillon cubes
- A handful fresh cilantro, chopped, to garnish
- 4 tablespoons coconut oil, divided
- 1 green chili, sliced

Method:

1. Make noodles of the zucchini using a spiralizer or julienne peeler.
2. Place a soup pot over medium-low heat. Add half the oil. When the oil is heated, add onions and sauté for a couple of minutes. Add salt, ginger and garlic and sauté for about 15 minutes. Stir occasionally.
3. Add curry powder, coconut milk, chili, water, salt and bouillon cubes and let it simmer for about 20 minutes.
4. Turn off the heat. Blend with an immersion blender until smooth.
5. Meanwhile, place a pan over medium flame. Add remaining oil. When the oil is heated, add tofu and cook until brown all over. Stir in the mushrooms and sauté for 3-4 minutes.
6. Add zucchini noodles mixture and cook for a couple of minutes.
7. Transfer into the soup pot. Heat thoroughly.
8. Divide into 4 soup bowls and serve garnished with cilantro.

Broccoli Cheese Soup

Number of servings: 2

Nutritional values per serving:

Calories – 560, Fat – 52 g, Total Carbohydrates – 12 g, Net Carbohydrates – 9.5 g, Protein – 15 g

Ingredients:

- 158.8 g /5.6 ounces broccoli, chopped
- 1 2/3 cups/710 ml heavy whipping cream
- ¾ cup/180 ml diced carrots
- 4 cloves garlic, minced
- Salt to taste
- Pepper to taste
- 158.8 g / 5.6 ounces cheddar cheese + extra to garnish if desired
- 1 ¼ cups diced onions
- ¾ cup/180 ml diced celery
- 1 ¾ tablespoons salted butter
- ½ teaspoon paprika or to taste, to garnish
- 1 ¾ cup/415 ml water

Method:

1. Place a soup pot over medium flame. Add butter. When it melts, add carrot, onions and celery and sauté until onion turns translucent.

2. Add broccoli and water and mix. Once it starts to boil, reduce the flame and simmer until vegetables are tender.

3. Add rest of the ingredients and stir. Turn off the heat.

4. Ladle into 4 soup bowls and serve.

Chapter Twelve: Ketogenic Lunch recipes

Collard Green Wraps

Number of servings: 2

Nutritional values per serving: 2 wraps with 2 tablespoons sauce per wrap

Calories – 330.68, Fat – 22.5 g, Total Carbohydrates – 19.08 g, Net Carbohydrates – 14.72 g, Protein – 13.96 g

Ingredients:

For Tzatziki Sauce:

- 2 cups/475 ml full-fat plain Greek yogurt
- 2 tablespoons white vinegar
- 1 small cucumber, grated, squeezed of excess moisture
- Salt to taste
- Pepper to taste
- 2 teaspoons garlic powder
- 4 tablespoons olive oil
- 4 tablespoons minced fresh dill

For wrap:

- 8 large collard green leaves, discard hard stems
- 1 medium red bell pepper, cut into thin strips
- 16 Kalamata olives, halved, pitted
- 16 cherry tomatoes, halved
- 2 medium cucumbers, cut into matchsticks
- 1 cup/240 ml diced onion
- 226.8 /8 ounces feta cheese, cut into 1 inch thick strips

Method:

1. To make Tzatziki sauce: Add all the ingredients for tzatziki sauce into a bowl and stir.
2. Cover and chill until use.
3. To make wraps: Spread the wraps on your countertop. Place 2 tablespoons tzatziki sauce on the wrap and spread it evenly, leaving aside the edges.
4. Scatter cucumber, onion, pepper, feta cheese, olives and tomatoes along the center of the wrap.
5. Wrap like a burrito and serve.

Grilled Cheese Sandwich

Number of servings: 2

Nutritional values per serving:

Calories – 803, Fat – 69.95 g, Total Carbohydrates – 18.14 g, Net Carbohydrates – 6.14 g, Protein – 25.84 g

Ingredients:

For bun:

- 8 large eggs
- 6 tablespoons psyllium husk powder
- 8 tablespoons butter, softened
- 8 tablespoons almond flour
- 2 teaspoons baking powder

Other ingredients:

- 4 tablespoons butter
- 226.8 g /8 ounces cheddar cheese

Method:

1. To make buns: Add all the ingredients for bun in a bowl and whisk until well incorporated.
2. Divide into 4 square, microwave safe bowls.

3. Microwave on high for 90 seconds. It the bun doesn't seem to be cooked, cook for a few seconds more (say 10 to 15 seconds).

4. Remove from the microwave and cool completely. Cut each bun into 2 halves, horizontally.

5. Divide cheese into 4 equal portions and place on the bottom half of the buns.

6. Cover with the top half of the buns.

7. Place a nonstick skillet over medium heat. Add ½ tablespoon butter. Place one sandwich on the pan. Spread ½ tablespoon butter on the top of the bun. Cook until it becomes brown on both sides.

8. Repeat the previous step and cook the remaining sandwiches.

Nori Wraps

Number of servings: 2

Nutritional values per serving:

Calories – 300, Fat – 23 g, Total Carbohydrates – 4 g, Net Carbohydrates – 2 g, Protein – 19 g

Ingredients:

- 12 pastured eggs
- 1 teaspoon salt
- 2 tablespoons butter or ghee
- 4 nori sheets
- 2 avocadoes, peeled, pitted, sliced

Method:

1. Add eggs and salt into a bowl and whisk well.

2. Place the nori sheets on your countertop.

3. Place a pan over medium heat. Add ½ tablespoon butter and melt. Tilt the pan so that the butter spreads.

4. Pour ¼ of the beaten eggs into the pan. Swirl the pan to spread the egg.

5. Cook until the egg is set. Carefully remove the omelet from the pan and place it directly on a sheet of nori.

6. Repeat the above steps and make the remaining omelets.

7. Spread avocado slices over the omelet.

8. Roll the nori sheets along with the omelet and avocado slices and place on a plate with the seam side facing down.

9. Cut each into 2 halves and serve.

Cheese Omelet

Number of servings: 2

Nutritional values per serving: ½ omelet

Calories – 897, Fat – 80 g, Total Carbohydrates – 4 g, Net Carbohydrates – 4 g, Protein – 40 g

Ingredients:

- 170 g / 6 ounces butter

- 397 g / 14 ounces cheddar cheese, shredded
- 12 eggs
- Salt to taste
- Pepper to taste

Method:

1. Add eggs and salt into a bowl and whisk well. Add salt, pepper and half the cheese and whisk again.
2. Place a nonstick pan over medium heat. Add half the butter. When butter melts, add half the egg and let it cook for a couple of minutes.
3. Lower the heat and cook until the omelet is set. Sprinkle half the cheese on one half of the omelet.
4. Fold the other half of the omelet over the cheese. Cook for a few seconds until cheese melts.
5. Remove onto a plate. Cut into 2 halves and serve.
6. Repeat steps 2-5 and make the remaining omelet.

Zucchini Pizza Boats

Number of servings: 2

Nutritional values per serving:

Calories – 693, Fat – 62 g, Total Carbohydrates – 5 g, Net Carbohydrates – 3 g, Protein – 27 g

Ingredients:

- 2 medium zucchinis
- ½ cup/120 ml olive oil
- 453.6 g / 16 ounces goat cheese
- 4 cloves garlic, peeled, thinly sliced
- 85 g /3 ounces baby spinach
- Salt and pepper to taste
- 4 tablespoons marinara sauce

Method:

1. Remove the seeds from the zucchini using a spoon. Do not discard the seeds and roughly chop them. So now you have your zucchini boats. Place on a baking sheet.
2. Place a skillet over medium flame. Add half the oil, add garlic and cook until light brown.
3. Stir in spinach and zucchini seeds and cook until tender. Add salt and pepper to taste. Turn off the heat.
4. Spread a tablespoon of marinara sauce on each zucchini half. Divide the spinach mixture among the boats.
5. Top with goat cheese.
6. Bake in a preheated oven at 375° F/190° C for around 25 minutes or until zucchini is tender.
7. Drizzle remaining oil on top. Sprinkle some pepper on top and serve.

Cheddar and Chive Soufflés

Number of servings: 2

Nutritional values per serving:

Calories – 212, Fat – 23.6 g, Total Carbohydrates – 3.32 g, Net Carbohydrates – 3.31 g, Protein – 14.02 g

Ingredients:

- ¼ cup/60 ml almond flour
- ½ teaspoon ground mustard
- ¼ teaspoon xanthan gum
- 6 tablespoons heavy cream
- 2 tablespoons fresh chives, chopped
- 1/8 teaspoon cream of tartar
- ½ teaspoon salt
- ¼ teaspoon pepper powder
- A pinch cayenne pepper
- 1 cup/240 ml cheddar cheese, shredded
- 3 large eggs, at room temperature, separated

Method:

1. Grease 4 ramekins with cooking spray or butter. Place the ramekins on a baking sheet.

2. Add almond flour, pepper, salt, mustard, cayenne pepper and xanthan gum into a bowl and mix well.

3. Add cheese, yolks, and chives and mix well.

4. Whip the whites with cream of tartar until stiff peaks are formed.

5. Add the whites into the bowl of dry ingredients. Fold gently until just mixed.

6. Divide and pour the mixture into the ramekins.

7. Bake in a preheated oven at 350° F/177° C for around 25 minutes or until the soufflés are well risen and golden brown on top.

8. Serve hot.

Spiralised Carrot and Zucchini Curry Noodles

Number of servings: 2

Nutritional values per serving:

Calories – 125, Fat – 6 g, Total Carbohydrates – 11 g, Net Carbohydrates – 7 g, Protein – 9 g

Ingredients:

- 2 medium zucchinis, trimmed
- 2 large carrots, trimmed, peeled

- 8 teaspoons red curry paste
- ½ cup/120 ml sliced scallions
- 4 hard boiled eggs, peeled, halved
- ¼ cup packed, chopped cilantro
- 4 lime wedges, to serve

Method:

1. Make noodles of the carrots and zucchini using a spiralizer fixed with blade D. cut the noodles into pieces of about 4-5 inches long.
2. Take 4 masons jar. Divide the curry paste among the 4 jars.
3. Next layer with equal amounts of scallions, cilantro, carrots, and zucchini. Finally place an egg and a lime wedge in each jar.
4. Fasten the lids and chill until use. It will last for about 2 days in the refrigerator.

Spiralised Daikon Miso Noodles with Tofu

Number of servings: 2

Nutritional values per serving:

Calories – 153, Fat – 8 g, Total Carbohydrates – 13 g, Net Carbohydrates – 8 g, Protein – 12 g

Ingredients:

- 2 daikon radishes, peeled, trimmed
- ½ cup/120 ml sliced scallions
- 2 bunches baby Bok Choy, trimmed, chopped
- 8 teaspoons miso paste
- 1 cup/240 ml cubed tofu, drained, pat dried
- 1 cup/240 ml sliced shiitake mushroom
- 4 teaspoons Sriracha sauce or any other hot sauce or chili paste
- 4 lime wedges, to serve

Method:

1. Make noodles of the daikon using a spiralizer fixed with blade D. Cut the noodles into pieces of about 4-5 inches long.
2. Take 4 masons jar. Divide the chili paste or hot sauce and miso paste among the 4 jars.
3. Next layer with equal amounts of - scallions, tofu, Bok Choy, mushroom and daikon. Place a lime wedge in each jar.
4. Fasten the lids and chill until use. It can last for 2 days in the refrigerator.

Braised Eggs with Leek and Za'atar

Number of servings: 2

Nutritional values per serving:

Calories – 223, Fat – 17 g, Total Carbohydrates – 9 g, Net Carbohydrates – NA, Protein – 10 g

Ingredients:

- 1 ½ tablespoons unsalted butter
- 353.33 g /12.5 ounces extra-large leeks, trimmed, cut into ¼ inch thick slices
- ½ teaspoon toasted, lightly crushed cumin seeds
- 2/3 cup/160 ml vegetable stock
- 4 large eggs
- ¾ tablespoon Za'atar
- 1 ½ tablespoons extra virgin olive oil, divided
- Freshly ground pepper to taste
- Kosher salt to taste
- 2 tablespoons chopped, preserved lemon (discard seeds)
- 78 g /4 2/3 ounces baby spinach
- 62.4 g /2.2 ounces feta, broken into ¾ inch pieces

Method:

1. Place a skillet over medium flame. Add butter and ½ tablespoon oil. When butter melts, stir in leeks, salt and a generous amount of pepper.
2. Sauté for 3 minutes.
3. Stir in cumin, stock and lemon and boil until the liquid in the pan is about 1/3 cup.

4. Add spinach and cook for a few seconds until it wilts. Lower the heat to medium heat.

5. Make 4 small wells (cavities) in the skillet (big enough for an egg to fit in).

6. Crack an egg in each well. Sprinkle salt and pepper.

7. Scatter feta cheese around the eggs. Cook until the whites are set.

8. Meanwhile, add remaining oil and za'atar. Drizzle oil mixture over the eggs and serve immediately.

Cauliflower Fried Rice

Number of servings: 2

Nutritional values per serving:

Calories – 127, Fat – 8 g, Total Carbohydrates –11 g, Net Carbohydrates – 6 g, Protein – 5 g

Ingredients:

- 1 ¾ tablespoons butter
- 1 red bell pepper, finely diced
- 1 medium head cauliflower, chopped into florets
- 1 medium onion, finely diced
- ¾ teaspoon toasted sesame oil
- 4 small cloves garlic, minced

- Salt to taste
- 2 small eggs
- Pepper to taste
- 4-5 teaspoons coconut aminos
- 2 medium green onions, sliced

Method:

1. Add the cauliflower florets to the food processor bowl and pulse until you get a rice like texture. Alternately, grate the cauliflower. You should have about 3 ¼ cups once grated.
2. Place a large skillet over medium high flame. Add ½ tablespoon butter. When the butter melts, add bell peppers and onions and sauté until onion turns golden brown. Add garlic and sauté for about a minute or so until fragrant.
3. Meanwhile, add eggs, salt and pepper in a bowl and mix well.
4. Move the vegetables to one side of the skillet. Add ½ tablespoon butter in the center of the pan.
5. Pour eggs in the center and scramble them. Move the eggs to one side of the pan.
6. Add remaining butter in the center of the pan. When butter melts, add cauliflower rice. Increase the heat to high heat and sauté the entire ingredients in the pan for about 5-6 minutes. Sprinkle salt and pepper and mix well. Remove from heat.
7. Add coconut aminos, green onion and sesame oil and toss well.
8. Serve hot.

Chapter Thirteen: Ketogenic Dinner Recipes

Vegetarian Coconut Red Curry

Number of servings: 2

Nutritional values per serving: Without cauliflower rice

Calories – 398, Fat – 40.73 g, Total Carbohydrates – 10.76 g, Net Carbohydrates – 7.86 g, Protein – 3.91 g

Ingredients:

- 2 cups/475 ml broccoli florets
- ½ cup/120 ml coconut oil
- 2 teaspoons minced ginger
- 2 teaspoons minced garlic
- 2 large handfuls spinach
- 1 small onion, chopped
- 4 teaspoons vegan fish sauce (can be found on Amazon)
- 2 tablespoons red curry paste
- 4 teaspoons soy sauce
- 1 cup/240 ml coconut cream or full-fat coconut milk

Method:

1. Place a skillet over medium flame. Add half the oil and once it gets heated, add onions and cook for a couple of minutes.

2. Add garlic and cook until brown.

3. Lower the heat and add broccoli. Mix well. Cover and cook for a few minutes until broccoli turns bright green in color.

4. Push the broccoli to one side of the pan.

5. Pour remaining oil in the center. Add red curry paste and cook for about a minute.

6. Mix the broccoli with the curry paste. Add spinach and mix well.

7. Add rest of the ingredients and mix well. Cook until slightly thick.

8. Serve over cauliflower rice.

Eggplant Lasagna

Number of servings: 2

Nutritional values per serving:

Calories – 474, Fat – 38 g, Total Carbohydrates – 14.1 g, Net Carbohydrates – 9 g, Protein – 20.7 g

Ingredients:

- 500 g /1 pound eggplant, slice into ½ inch thick slices
- 220 g /7.7 ounces fresh spinach

- 4 large eggs
- 4 tablespoons ghee, melted
- ½ cup/120 ml + 1/3 cup/80 ml grated mozzarella cheese
- ¾ cup/180 ml feta cheese, grated
- 5 ½ tablespoons grated parmesan cheese
- 1 tablespoon chopped fresh oregano
- ½ cup/120 ml + 2 tablespoons marinara sauce
- 1 tablespoon chopped fresh basil
- Salt to taste

Method:

1. Place the sliced eggplant on a baking sheet. Brush liberally with ghee. Sprinkle a little salt.
2. Bake in a preheated oven at 400° F/205° C for about 20 minutes. Remove from the oven and set aside.
3. Meanwhile, place a pot of water over high flame. When it boils add the spinach and cook for a minute.
4. Drain the water and immediately place the spinach in a bowl of chilled water. Let it remain in it for a few minutes. Drain by placing in a colander. Squeeze out the excess moisture from spinach.
5. Place a skillet over medium heat. Add a little ghee and allow it to melt.
6. Beat an egg at a time. Add a pinch of salt and whisk again. Pour into the skillet
7. Swirl the pan to get a thin omelet.

8. Cook for a couple of minutes until the top is set. Gently slide on to a plate.

9. Repeat the above 3 steps with the remaining eggs.

10. To assemble: Take a small square or rectangular baking dish.

11. Place 2 omelets on the bottom of the dish.

12. Spread half the marinara sauce over the omelets. Place half the eggplant slices over it. Next, sprinkle half the mozzarella cheese followed by half the spinach. Sprinkle half the feta cheese.

13. Place 2 omelets over the feta layer.

14. Repeat step 12.

15. Sprinkle parmesan cheese on top.

16. Bake in a preheated oven at 400° F/205° C for about 20-30 minutes or until the top is golden brown.

17. Remove from the oven and let it cool for a few minutes.

18. Serve hot or warm.

Vegan Zucchini Lasagna

Number of servings: 2

Nutritional values per serving:

Calories – 338, Fat – 34 g, Total Carbohydrates – 10 g, Net Carbohydrates – 5 g, Protein – 4.7 g

Ingredients:

For vegan ricotta cheese:

- 1 1/3 cups/310 ml raw macadamia nuts or soaked blanched almonds
- ½ cup/120 ml finely chopped basil
- 2 teaspoons lemon juice
- Salt to taste
- Pepper to taste
- 1 tablespoon vegan parmesan cheese + optional extra to serve
- 2 ½ teaspoons nutritional yeast
- ½ teaspoon dried oregano
- 1 teaspoon extra virgin olive oil (optional)
- 2-3 tablespoons water or more if required

Other ingredients:

- 1 1/3 zucchinis, thinly sliced with a mandolin slicer
- 12.5 ounces marinara sauce

Method:

- To make ricotta cheese: Place macadamia nuts into the food processor and process until finely ground.
- Add rest of the ingredients and process until well incorporated. Taste and add more seasonings, lemon juice and nutritional yeast if required.
- To assemble: Take a small square or rectangular baking dish.
- Spread some marinara sauce on the bottom of the dish.

- Place a layer of zucchini. Next spread some ricotta mixture over it. Spread it evenly and in a thin layer. Spread a layer of marinara sauce.
- Repeat the previous step until all the ricotta, zucchini and marinara sauce is used up.
- Sprinkle vegan parmesan cheese on top.
- Cover the dish with foil.
- Bake in a preheated oven at 375º F for about 35-40 minutes. Uncover and bake for another 15 minutes.
- Remove from the oven and cool for 10 minutes.
- Garnish with extra vegan parmesan cheese if using and serve.

Keto White Pizza

Number of servings: 2

Nutritional values per serving:

Calories – 1090, Fat – 100 g, Total Carbohydrates – 11 g, Net Carbohydrates – 8 g, Protein – 36 g

Ingredients:

For crust:

- 4 eggs
- 1 ½ cups/335 ml almond flour
- 2 teaspoons baking powder
- 1 cup/240 ml mayonnaise or crème fraiche

- 2 tablespoons ground psyllium husk powder
- 1 teaspoon salt

For topping:

- 1 cup/240 ml sour cream or crème fraiche
- 113.4 g /4 ounces parmesan cheese, grated
- Pepper to taste
- 1 ½ cups/335 ml shredded cheese
- 2 teaspoons minced fresh rosemary or teaspoon dried rosemary

Method:

1. Preheat the oven at 350° F/177° C.
2. To make crust: Add mayonnaise and eggs into a bowl and whisk well.
3. Add rest of the ingredients and mix well.
4. Line a baking sheet with parchment paper.
5. Place dough on the parchment paper.
6. Grease your rolling pin lightly with some oil and roll the mixture until it is about ½ inch in thickness.
7. Bake at 350° F/177° C for about 10 minutes or until light brown.
8. Remove the baking sheet from the oven.
9. For topping: Flip the crust on the baking sheet.
10. Spoon sour cream on the crust. Spread it evenly. Sprinkle cheese, rosemary and pepper on top.

11. Bake in a preheated oven at 375° F/190° C for about 6-10 minutes. Keep a watch over the pizza so that it does not get burnt.

12. Sprinkle parmesan cheese on top.

13. Cut into 4 wedges and serve.

Grilled Veggie Plate

Number of servings: 2

Nutritional values per serving:

Calories – 1013, Fat – 99 g, Total Carbohydrates – 15 g, Net Carbohydrates – 9 g, Protein – 21 g

Ingredients:

- 1 zucchini, cut into ½ inch thick slices lengthwise
- 1 medium eggplant, cut into ½ inch thick slices, lengthwise
- ½ cup/120 ml olive oil
- 20 black olives
- 1 cup/240 ml mayonnaise
- Salt to taste
- Pepper to taste
- Juice of a lemon
- ¼ cup almonds

- 56.7 g /2 ounces leafy greens

Method:

1. Sprinkle salt on either side of the zucchini and eggplant slices and place in a colander for 5 minutes.

2. Set the oven to broil mode and preheat the oven.

3. Dry the zucchini and eggplant slices by patting with paper towels.

4. Place a parchment paper on the baking sheet. Place the zucchini and eggplant slices on baking sheet.

5. Brush oil over the slices. Sprinkle pepper.

6. Broil for about 15-20 minutes. Flip sides halfway through broiling.

7. Divide into 4 serving plates. Drizzle oil and lemon juice over the slices.

8. Divide equally olives, almonds and leafy greens among the plate. Place ¼ cup mayonnaise in each plate and serve. Roast the almonds if desired.

Zucchini "Meatballs"

Number of servings: 2

Nutritional values per serving: 1 meatball without serving options

Calories – 71, Fat – 6.6 g, Total Carbohydrates – 2.7 g, Net Carbohydrates – 1.1 g, Protein – 1.7 g

Ingredients:

- 1/3 cup/80 ml shredded (squeezed of excess moisture) zucchini

- 1/8 teaspoon salt or to taste
- 1 teaspoon Italian seasoning
- 1 teaspoon psyllium husk
- 1 teaspoon dried oregano
- A pinch red pepper flakes
- 1/3 cup/80 ml chopped or ground walnuts
- 1/8 teaspoon granulated garlic

Serving options:

- Zucchini noodles or shirataki noodles
- Marinara sauce or any other keto-friendly sauce of your choice

Method:

1. Preheat the oven at 375° F/190° C
2. Place a sheet of parchment paper on a baking sheet.
3. Add zucchini, salt and walnuts into a bowl and mix well. Set aside for 8-10 minutes.
4. Add rest of the ingredients and mix well.
5. Divide the mixture into 4 equal portions and shape into balls. Place on prepared baking sheet.
6. Bake for about 6-10 minutes.
7. Serve with suggested serving options.

Spicy Almond Tofu

Number of servings: 2

Nutritional values per serving:

Calories – Fat – 29 g, Total Carbohydrates – 10 g, Net Carbohydrates – 5 g, Protein – 24 g

Ingredients:

- 2 packages firm tofu or extra firm tofu
- 4 tablespoons liquid aminos
- ½ teaspoon onion powder
- ½ teaspoon garlic powder
- ½ teaspoon paprika
- ½ teaspoon chili flakes
- Salt to taste
- Pepper to taste
- ½ teaspoon Himalayan pink salt
- 4 tablespoons water
- 2 tablespoons sesame seeds, divided
- 2 teaspoons sesame oil
- 2 tablespoons coconut oil
- 4 tablespoons green chili sauce

- ¼ cup sliced almonds
- Steamed broccoli to serve

Method:

1. Place tofu on paper towels. Place a heavy skillet over the tofu to drain out excess moisture. Let it remain like this for about an hour.
2. Chop tofu into cubes.
3. Place a skillet over high heat. Add coconut oil. When the oil is heated, add tofu and sauté until golden brown.
4. Add almonds and cook for 2 minutes. Add rest of the ingredients except ½ tablespoon sesame seeds and sesame oil and cook until dry.
5. Divide steamed broccoli into 4 bowls. Place tofu on top. Drizzle sesame oil over it. Sprinkle remaining sesame seeds on top and serve.

Portabella Pizza

Number of servings: 2

Nutritional values per serving: 4 mushrooms

Calories – 126, Fat – 7.1 g, Total Carbohydrates – 9.6 g, Net Carbohydrates – 7.4 g, Protein – 7.7 g

Ingredients:

- 16 medium to large Portabella mushrooms or large mushroom caps, discard stems
- 2 medium green peppers, chopped

- 2 medium yellow onions, chopped
- 4 cloves garlic, peeled, minced
- Pepper to taste
- Salt to taste
- 2 cups/475 ml marinara sauce or any other keto-friendly pizza sauce
- ½ cup/120 ml grated parmesan cheese
- 4 tablespoons olive oil
- 2 cups/475 ml shredded part-skim mozzarella cheese

Method:

1. Place mushroom caps on a baking sheet, with the stem side facing up.
2. Bake in a preheated oven at 375° F for about 10 minutes.
3. Heat a skillet over medium flame and add some oil. When the oil gets hot, add onion and green pepper and sauté until onion turns translucent.
4. Add garlic, salt and pepper and sauté for a few seconds until aromatic. Turn off the heat.
5. Remove the baking sheet from the oven and dab the mushrooms with paper towels.
6. Spread 2 tablespoons sauce in each mushroom cap (on the stem part).
7. Divide the onion mixture among the mushroom caps.
8. Sprinkle 2 tablespoons mozzarella cheese on each cap. Sprinkle ½ tablespoon parmesan cheese on each cap.
9. Bake in a preheated oven at 375° F/190° C for about 10 minutes or until cheese melts and is bubbling.

Lo Mein

Number of servings: 2

Nutritional values per serving:

Calories – 195, Fat – 13.9 g, Total Carbohydrates – 8.9 g, Net Carbohydrates – 4.4 g, Protein – 5.1 g

Ingredients:

- 4 packages kelp noodles
- 4 cups/950 ml frozen broccoli florets
- ½ cup/120 ml shredded or julienned carrots

For the sauce:

- 8 tablespoons tamari or soy sauce
- 2 teaspoons ground ginger
- 1 teaspoon Sriracha sauce
- 4 tablespoons sesame oil
- 2 teaspoons garlic powder

Method:

1. Soak the kelp noodles in a bowl of water for a while. Drain and set aside.
2. To make sauce: Place a saucepan over medium-low heat. Add all the ingredients for the sauce into the saucepan and heat.
3. When the sauce is heated, add noodles and mix well. Add some water if desired so that the mixture is not very dry.

4. Cook until the noodles are soft. Remove from heat. Let it rest for a couple of minutes.

5. Divide among 4 bowls and serve.

Pumpkin Cheddar Risotto

Number of servings: 2

Nutritional values per serving:

Calories – 223, Fat – 16.3 g, Total Carbohydrates – 9.9 g, Net Carbohydrates – 6.5 g, Protein – 9.4 g

Ingredients:

- 1 small onion, chopped
- 2 ½ teaspoons paprika or to taste
- 2/3 cup/160 ml pumpkin puree or butternut squash puree
- 453.6 g /16 ounces cauliflower
- 113.4 g /4 ounces cheddar cheese, shredded
- 2 ¾ tablespoons butter
- Pepper to taste
- Salt to taste
- 1 cup/240 ml pumpkin or butternut squash puree
- 1/3 cup/80 ml heavy cream (optional)

Method:

1. Add the cauliflower florets to the food processor bowl and pulse until you get a rice like texture. Alternately, grate the cauliflower.

2. Place a large saucepan over medium heat. Add butter. When the butter melts, add onion and sauté until it becomes translucent. Add paprika, salt and pepper and stir for 5-6 seconds.

3. Add heavy cream if using, pumpkin puree and cauliflower and mix well. Lower the heat to low heat.

4. Cover with a lid and simmer for 15 minutes or until the cauliflower turns soft. Stir a couple of times while it is cooking. Taste and adjust the seasoning as necessary.

5. Remove from heat. Add cheddar cheese and stir.

6. Serve hot.

Chapter Fourteen: Ketogenic Side Dish Recipes

Zucchini Noodles with Avocado Sauce

Number of servings: 2

Nutritional values per serving:

Calories – 313, Fat – 26.8 g, Total Carbohydrates – 18.7 g, Net Carbohydrates – 9 g, Protein – 6.8 g

Ingredients:

- 2 zucchinis, trimmed
- 2/3 cup/160 ml water
- 4 tablespoons lemon juice
- 24 cherry tomatoes, sliced
- 2 ½ cups basil
- ½ cup/120 ml pine nuts
- 2 avocadoes, peeled, pitted, chopped

Method:

1. Using a spiralizer, make noodles of the zucchini. You can also use a julienne peeler to make the noodles.

2. Place in a bowl. Add tomatoes and toss well.

3. Add rest of the ingredients in a blender and blend well until it becomes smooth. Pour over the zucchini. Fold gently and serve.

4. You can save the leftovers in an airtight container in the refrigerator.

Broccoli and Cheese Fritters

Number of servings: 2

Nutritional values per serving: 1 fritter without sauce

Calories – 78, Fat – 5.8 g, Total Carbohydrates – 3.78 g, Net Carbohydrates – 1.3 g, Protein – 4.6 g

Nutritional values per serving: 1 fritter with sauce

Calories – 103.9, Fat – 8.35 g, Total Carbohydrates – 4.37 g, Net Carbohydrates – 1.89 g, Protein – 4.6 g

Ingredients:

For fritters:

- 3 tablespoons almond flour
- 1 ounce fresh broccoli
- 1 small egg

- Salt to taste
- Pepper to taste
- 2 tablespoons flaxseed meal + extra to dredge
- 1 ounce mozzarella cheese
- ½ teaspoon baking powder
- Oil, as required, to fry

For sauce:

- 1 tablespoon mayonnaise
- 1 teaspoon lemon juice
- 1 tablespoon chopped fresh dill
- Salt to taste
- Pepper to taste

Method:

1. Place broccoli in the food processor and process until finely chopped.
2. Place the rest of the ingredients and process until well combined.
3. Divide the mixture into 4 equal portions and shape into balls. Dredge in flaxseed meal.
4. Fry the fritters in a deep fryer until golden brown in color.
5. Remove the fritters and place on a plate lined with paper towels.
6. Meanwhile, make the sauce by mixing together all the ingredients for the sauce in a bowl.
7. Serve fritters with sauce.

Keto Bread

Number of servings: 2

Nutritional values per serving: 1 mini loaf

Calories – 196, Fat – 16.8 g, Total Carbohydrates – 3.8 g, Net Carbohydrates – 2 g, Protein – 8 g

Ingredients:

- 4 large eggs
- 4 tablespoons olive oil
- 4 tablespoons coconut flour
- 4 tablespoons almond flour or hazelnut flour
- ½ teaspoon salt or to taste
- 4 tablespoons milk
- 1 teaspoon baking powder

Optional ingredients:

- 4 tablespoons minced fresh herbs of your choice or minced scallions
- 1 cup/240 ml grated cheese

Method:

1. Add all the ingredients into a bowl and mix until well incorporated.
2. Stir in the cheese and scallions.

3. Divide the mixture into 4 tall microwave safe mugs. Tap the mugs on the countertop a few times.

4. Place in the microwave and cook on high for 90 seconds.

5. When the bread is ready, carefully invert on a plate.

6. Cut into slices and serve. Toast the bread slices if desired.

Creamed Spinach

Number of servings: 2

Nutritional values per serving: 1 cup/240 ml

Calories – 548, Fat – 54 g, Total Carbohydrates – 10 g, Net Carbohydrates – 8 g, Protein – 8 g

Ingredients:

- 6 tablespoons butter
- 567 g /20 ounces baby spinach, chopped
- 170 g / 6 ounces cream cheese, cut into small pieces
- ½ teaspoon sea salt
- Parmesan cheese, grated, to top (optional)
- 8 cloves garlic, peeled, minced
- 1 cup/240 ml heavy cream
- 2 teaspoons Italian seasoning

- ½ teaspoon pepper

Method:

1. Place a wok over medium flame. Add the butter and let it melt. Stir in the garlic and cook for a few seconds until it becomes aromatic.

2. Stir in the spinach and cover with a lid. Cook until it wilts. Stir frequently.

3. Add rest of the ingredients and mix well. Cook until cream cheese melts and the mixture thickens. Stir frequently.

4. Garnish with parmesan and serve.

Baked Cauliflower Casserole with Goat Cheese

Number of servings: 2

Nutritional values per serving:

Calories – 127.7, Fat – 6.4 g, Total Carbohydrates – 16 g, Net Carbohydrates – 10.8 g, Protein – 5.7 g

Ingredients:

- 4 cups/950 ml cauliflower florets
- ¾ teaspoon dried oregano
- Pepper to taste
- Salt to taste
- 3 teaspoons olive oil

- 42.5 g / 1 ½ ounces goat cheese, crumbled

For sauce:

- ¾ teaspoon olive oil
- 530.13 g / 18.7 ounces canned, crushed tomatoes
- Salt to taste
- 2 cloves garlic, peeled, minced
- 1 bay leaf
- 3 tablespoons minced flat-leaf parsley

Method:

1. Place cauliflower in a baking dish. Drizzle some oil on it and sprinkle with salt, pepper and oregano over it and toss well. Spread it evenly.
2. Bake it in a preheated oven at 425° F/220° C for about 25 minutes or until fork tender. Stir a couple of times while baking.
3. Remove the baking dish from the oven and spread marinara sauce over it.
4. Sprinkle goat cheese on top. Bake for another 20 minutes or until cheese melts.
5. Meanwhile, make the sauce as follows: Place a nonstick pan over medium heat. Add oil. Once the oil gets heated, toss the garlic and sauté until aromatic.
6. Add tomatoes and bay leaf and mix well.
7. When it boils, lower the flame and simmer for 12-15 minutes.
8. Discard the bay leaf. Add salt and parsley and stir.
9. Serve casserole with sauce.

Creamy Greek Zucchini Patties

Number of servings: 2

Nutritional values per serving: 3 patties

Calories – 159, Fat – 15 g, Total Carbohydrates – 6 g, Net Carbohydrates – NA, Protein – 6 g

Ingredients:

- 453.6 g / 1 pound zucchini, trimmed, grated
- A large handful mixture of fresh dill, mint and parsley
- ½ cup/120 ml crumbled feta cheese
- ½ teaspoon fine grain sea salt
- 1 ½ tablespoons olive oil, divided
- 1 large egg
- ½ cup/120 ml almond meal
- ½ teaspoon ground cumin
- Pepper to taste

Method:

1. Toss zucchini with some salt and place in a colander. Set aside for an hour.
2. Squeeze the zucchini of excess moisture. Place in a bowl.
3. Add all the ingredients except oil into the bowl of zucchini and mix well. Chill for about 30 minutes.

4. Divide the mix into 12 portions and shape into patties.

5. Place a large nonstick pan over medium-high heat. Add about half the oil. Swirl the pan to spread the oil. Place a few patties on the pan and cook until it becomes golden on both sides.

6. Remove onto a plate.

7. Repeat steps 5-6 and fry the remaining patties.

Cheesy Ranch Roasted Broccoli

Number of servings: 2

Nutritional values per serving:

Calories – 135, Fat – 11 g, Total Carbohydrates – NA, Net Carbohydrates – 3 g, Protein – 4 g

Ingredients:

- 2 2/3 cups/910 g broccoli florets
- 1/3 cup/43 g shredded sharp cheddar cheese
- Salt to taste
- Pepper to taste
- 3 tablespoons heavy whipping cream
- 3 tablespoons keto-friendly ranch dressing

Method:

1. Add all the ingredients into an oven-proof casserole dish and mix well. Spread it evenly.

2. Bake in a preheated oven at 375° F/190° C for about 40 minutes or until tender. Stir a couple of times while baking.

3. Remove from the oven and let it sit for a couple of minutes before serving.

Wilted Beet Greens with Goat Cheese and Pine Nuts

Number of servings: 2

Nutritional values per serving:

Calories – 215, Fat – 18 g, Total Carbohydrates – NA, Net Carbohydrates – 3.5 g, Protein – 10 g

Ingredients:

- 8 cups/340 g beet greens, chopped
- 2 tablespoons balsamic vinegar
- 4 ounces goat cheese, crumbled
- 6 teaspoons olive oil, divided
- ¼ cup/32 g toasted pine nuts

Method:

1. Place a large skillet over medium flame. Add some oil and once the oil heats, add the beet greens and sauté until it wilts.

2. Get it off heat. Add salt and pepper and mix well.

3. Whisk together in a bowl, vinegar and remaining oil.

4. Place equal quantities of beet greens on 4 serving plates. Scatter pine nuts and goat cheese over the greens. Drizzle the dressing on top and serve.

Chapter Fifteen: Ketogenic Dessert Recipes

Raspberry Lemon Popsicles

Number of servings: 2

Nutritional values per serving:

Calories – 151, Fat – 16 g, Total Carbohydrates – 3.3 g, Net Carbohydrates – 2 g, Protein – 0.5 g

Ingredients:

- 66 g /2.34 ounces raspberries
- 3 tablespoons coconut oil
- 3 tablespoons sour cream
- ¼ teaspoon +1/8 teaspoon guar gum
- 1 tablespoon lemon juice
- 2/3 cup/160 ml coconut milk
- 3 tablespoons heavy cream
- 15 drops liquid stevia or to taste

Method:

1. Toss all ingredients in a blender and blend until it becomes smooth.
2. Place a wire mesh strainer over a bowl. Pour the blended mixture into the strainer. Discard the solids remaining in the strainer.
3. Pour the strained mixture into 4 popsicle molds. Insert the sticks.
4. Freeze until set.
5. To serve. Dip the molds in hot water for a few seconds to remove the popsicle. This will help remove the popsicle easily.
6. Serve.

Strawberry Popsicle

Number of servings: 2

Nutritional values per serving:

Calories – 234, Fat – 22.5 g, Total Carbohydrates – 4.5 g, Net Carbohydrates – 3.75 g, Protein – 2.6 g

Ingredients:

- 1 cup/240 ml strawberries, fresh or frozen
- ½ cup/120 ml coconut milk or heavy whipping cream
- 1 teaspoon vanilla extract or ½ teaspoon vanilla powder
- ½ cup/120 ml creamed coconut milk or mascarpone cheese
- 2 tablespoons erythritol or swerve sweetener or stevia to taste

- 5-8 drops stevia drops (optional)

Method:

1. Add all the ingredients into the blender and blend it until it becomes smooth.

2. Pour into 4 popsicle molds. Insert the sticks.

3. Freeze until set.

4. To serve. Dip the molds in hot water for a few seconds to remove the popsicle. This will help remove the popsicle easily.

5. Serve.

Avocado Popsicle with Coconut & Lime

Number of servings: 2

Nutritional values per serving:

Calories – 219, Fat – 21 g, Total Carbohydrates – 8 g, Net Carbohydrates – 4 g, Protein – 2 g

Ingredients:

- 1 1/3 avocadoes, pitted, peeled, chopped
- 3 tablespoons erythritol
- 1 cup/240 ml coconut milk
- 1 1/3 tablespoons lime juice

Method:

1. Add all the ingredients into the blender and blend until smooth.
2. Pour into 4 popsicle molds. Insert the sticks.
3. Freeze until set.
4. To serve. Dip the molds in a bowl of hot water for a few seconds to remove the popsicle. This will help remove the Popsicle easily.
5. Serve.

Pumpkin pie

Number of servings: 2

Nutritional values per serving:

Calories – 490, Fat – 48 g, Total Carbohydrates – 13 g, Net Carbohydrates – 6 g, Protein – 7 g

Ingredients:

For filling:

- 170 g /6 ounces pumpkin, peeled, deseeded, chopped
- ½ cup/120 ml heavy whipping cream
- 1 teaspoon pumpkin pie spice
- 2 tablespoons butter
- 1 egg

- A small pinch salt

For pie crust:

- 3 tablespoons butter, at room temperature
- 3 tablespoons hazelnut flour
- 6 tablespoons coconut flour
- 1/8 teaspoon vanilla extract
- 1/8 teaspoon ground cinnamon

For topping:

- ½ teaspoon lemon zest, grated
- ¾ teaspoon heavy whipping cream

Method:

1. Grease 4 small springform pans (3 inches each) or 1 bigger springform pan (8 inches) with some butter. Set aside.
2. To make crust: Add all the ingredients for pie crust into a bowl and mix until smooth dough is formed.
3. Press the dough into the prepared pans / pan. Press it on the bottom as well as the sides of the pan/ pans.
4. Bake in a preheated oven at 350° F/177° C for 10 minutes if you are using the 3 inch pans and 15 minutes if you are using the bigger pan.
5. To make filling: Place a pan over medium heat. Add pumpkin, butter and cream into a pan.
6. When it boils, lower the heat to low and cook until pumpkin is softened and the mixture is nearly dry. Stir frequently.

7. Turn off the heat and cool for 10-12 minutes.

8. Add pumpkin pie spice, egg, and salt into the pan. Blend with an immersion blender until smooth.

9. Spread this mixture over the baked crust/crusts.

10. Place the pan/pans in the oven.

11. Bake for another 15-20 minutes for the 3 inch pans or for about 30 minutes for the bigger pan or until the filling is set. If you find that the edges are burning, cover aluminum foil all around the edges of the pie crust or lower the temperature of the oven.

12. Remove from the oven and cool for some time.

13. To make topping: Add cream into a bowl. Beat with an electric hand mixer until soft peaks are formed. Add lemon zest and mix well. Cut into 4 wedges for the bigger pie. Spread the topping over the filling.

14. Serve.

Mascarpone Cheese Mousse and Berries

Number of servings: 2

Nutritional values per serving: With berries

Calories – 165, Fat – 15.9 g, Total Carbohydrates – 3.8 g, Net Carbohydrates – 3.2 g, Protein – 1.9 g

Nutritional values per serving: Without berries

Calories – 153, Fat – 15.8 g, Total Carbohydrates – 0.9 g, Net Carbohydrates – 0 g, Protein – 1.7 g

Ingredients:

- 2.6 ounces mascarpone cheese
- ¼ teaspoon vanilla stevia drops or to taste
- 1/3 cup/80 ml whipping cream
- 1/3 pint berries (mixture of blueberries and strawberries) (optional)

Method:

1. Add mascarpone cheese, sweetener and cream into a bowl and beat with an electric hand mixer until stiff peaks are formed.
2. Spoon into cups and serve.
3. If using berries, layer with mousse and berries and serve.

Chocolate Peanut Butter Hearts

Number of servings: 2

Nutritional values per serving:

Calories – 95, Fat – 6 g, Total Carbohydrates – 7 g, Net Carbohydrates – 2 g, Protein – 5 g

Ingredients:

- 6 ½ tablespoons smooth peanut butter, unsweetened
- 3 ½ tablespoons coconut flour

- 2 ½ tablespoons sticky keto-friendly sweetener of your choice
- ½ cup/120 ml chocolate chips

Method:

1. Place a sheet of parchment paper on a plate.
2. Add peanut butter and sticky sweetener into a glass bowl and microwave it on high for 60-70 seconds or until well melted. Stir every 20 seconds.
3. Add coconut flour and mix well. Set aside for 10 minutes.
4. Divide the mix into 4 equal portions and shape into balls. Flatten them slightly and shape into hearts.
5. Melt the chocolate using a chocolate melter or a double boiler.
6. Dip the peanut butter hearts in the chocolate and lift with a fork.
7. Place on the prepared plate. Chill until the chocolate sets.
8. Serve.

Keto Ice Cream

Number of servings: 2

Nutritional values per serving:

Calories – 347, Fat – 36 g, Total Carbohydrates – 3 g, Net Carbohydrates – 3 g, Protein – 2 g

Ingredients:

- 1 ½ tablespoons butter

- 3 tablespoons powdered erythritol
- 2 tablespoons MCT oil or MCT oil powder
- 1 ½ cups/335 ml heavy cream, divided
- ½ teaspoon vanilla extract
- 1 small vanilla bean, seeds scraped (optional)

Method:

1. Add butter and 1 cup/240 ml heavy cream in a pan. Heat the pan over medium flame.
2. When it starts to boil, lower the flame and let it simmer for about 15-20 minutes or until it is half its original quantity. Stir occasionally.
3. Transfer into a bowl and set aside to cool completely.
4. Add vanilla extract and vanilla seeds if using. Mix well.
5. Add remaining cream and whisk well.
6. Chill for an hour in the freezer.
7. Pour the mix into an ice cream maker and let it churn. Follow the instructions on the ice cream maker to make the perfect ice cream.
8. Serve right out of the ice cream maker for soft serve ice cream. For firm ice cream, transfer into a freezer safe container and freeze until firm.
9. If you do not have an ice cream maker, after step 5, pour into a freezer safe container and freeze until firm. Stir every 30 minutes until firm.
10. Divide into 4 bowls and serve.

Butter Pecan Ice Cream

Number of servings: 2

Nutritional values per serving:

Calories – 302, Fat – 32 g, Total Carbohydrates – 2 g, Net Carbohydrates – NA, Protein – 2 g

Ingredients:

- 2 tablespoons butter
- ¼ cup swerve confectioners sweetener
- 1 egg yolk
- ½ tablespoon chocZero maple pecan sweetener or sweetener of your choice
- 1 tablespoon toasted, chopped pecans
- 1 cup/240 ml heavy cream
- 1/8 teaspoon salt
- 1 teaspoon maple extract
- ½ tablespoon MCT oil

Method:

1. Add butter, cream, salt and sweetener into a small saucepan. Place the saucepan over low heat. When the mixture melts, turn off the heat. Do not heat for long.
2. Beat yolk in a bowl. Add a spoonful of the cream mixture and mix well.
3. Repeat adding the cream mixture 2 to 3 times.

4. Pour the yolk mixture into the saucepan. Place the saucepan over low heat.

5. Stir constantly until thick and temperature of the mixture is 175° F.

6. Turn off the heat. Pour into a bowl. Chill for 30 minutes.

7. Stir in maple extract, MCT oil and choczero maple pecan sweetener.

8. Pour the mix into an ice cream maker and let it churn. Follow the instructions on the ice cream maker to make the perfect ice cream.

9. Transfer into a freezer safe container. Sprinkle pecans on top and freeze until firm.

10. If you do not have an ice cream maker, after step 7, pour into a freezer safe container and freeze until firm. Stir every 30 minutes until firm. Sprinkle pecans when you stir for the last time.

11. Divide into 4 bowls and serve.

No Bake Low-Carb Lemon Strawberry Cheesecake Treats

Number of servings: 2

Nutritional values per serving:

Calories – 474, Fat – 48.2 g, Total Carbohydrates – 5.7 g, Net Carbohydrates – 5.3 g, Protein – 4.5 g

Ingredients:

- 177.4 /6 ounces cream cheese, softened
- 2/3 cup/160 ml swerve sweetener
- Zest of 2 lemons, grated

- 1 ½ cups/335 ml heavy whipping cream
- 4 teaspoons lemon extract
- 4 large strawberries, chopped

Method:

1. Add cream cheese, whipping cream and sweetener into a mixing bowl. Whip on high speed until fluffy.
2. Add lemon extract and some of the lemon zest and whip again until well incorporated.
3. Take 4 jars. Divide half the cream cheese mixture among the 4 jars.
4. Divide half the strawberries among the jars. Divide remaining cream cheese mixture and layer over the strawberries.
5. Sprinkle remaining strawberries and lemon zest on top and serve.

Pumpkin Spice Crème Brulee

Number of servings: 2

Nutritional values per serving:

Calories – 460, Fat – 49 g, Total Carbohydrates – NA, Net Carbohydrates – 5 g, Protein – 5g

Ingredients:

- 2 cups/475 ml heavy cream
- 4 egg yolks

- 4 tablespoons erythritol + 4 teaspoons extra for sprinkling
- 4 tablespoons pumpkin puree
- 2 teaspoons pumpkin pie spice

Method:

1. Place a heavy bottomed pan over low heat. Add cream and heat.
2. Once it starts bubbling, add pumpkin pie spice and stir. Remove from heat. Cover and set aside for 5 minutes.
3. Whisk the yolks until pale yellow in color.
4. Add about a tablespoon of the cream mixture to the eggs and whisk constantly. Continue this process until all the cream is added.
5. Add pumpkin puree and whisk again. Add erythritol and stir until it dissolves completely.
6. Transfer into 4 ramekins. Take a large baking dish. Pour enough hot water to cover 1 inch from the bottom of the dish.
7. Place the ramekins inside the baking dish.
8. Bake in a preheated oven at 300°F for about 45 minutes or until set. It will be jiggling slightly.
9. Remove from the oven and cool. Refrigerate for 5-6 hours.
10. Sprinkle 1 teaspoon erythritol on top of each ramekin.
11. Using a culinary torch, caramelize the tops or broil for a couple of minutes.
12. Serve chilled or at room temperature.

Chapter Sixteen: Tips To Stay Motivated

Getting started with a new diet can be overwhelming. However, there are a few things you can do to ensure that your motivation levels don't falter. In this section, you will learn about some practical tips which you can use to ensure that you stay motivated while following the keto diet.

Before you get started with the diet, make sure that you take some time and establish certain goals yourself. Why do you want to follow the vegetarian keto diet? Make sure that the goals you are setting for yourself are specific, measurable, attainable, realistic, and time bound (S.M.A.R.T). If the goal you set doesn't meet any of these criteria, the chances of giving up on the diet increase exponentially.

You must understand that making any dietary changes is a significant change for your body. As with any change, it will certainly take your body some time to get used to the new diet. So, be patient with yourself and give yourself the time required to get accustomed to the new diet. Another thing that you must keep in mind is that you need to follow this diet for a while before you can see any improvement. Don't expect any miraculous changes overnight. If you put in the necessary hard work and make a conscious effort, you will see an improvement in your overall health as well as weight.

You cannot attain success without facing certain obstacles. The only thing that matters is your attitude while dealing with such obstacles and setbacks. If you start thinking of them as failures, you will want to give up on your diet. There will be times when you might feel like giving up on your diet and bingeing on some unhealthy food that you must not. You might give up on your diet and indulge yourself also. If that happens, treat it as an isolated incident and not as a failure. Don't try to be a perfectionist when it comes to dieting.

You need to reward yourself whenever you attain any of your goals. The reward you set for yourself doesn't have to be anything big. Something as simple as buying the nail polish that you wanted or going for a massage. You must not only celebrate yourself but must also reward yourself for the effort you put in. If you stick to your diet, you certainly deserve a reward. If you keep rewarding yourself whenever you attain a goal, it gives your morale the boost it needs to keep going.

Keep in mind that following the keto diet isn't a temporary solution, but it is a lifelong process. If you want to lose weight and maintain weight loss, then you must come up with a maintenance plan for this diet in the long run. It means that you must have a maintenance plan in mind. It is better to develop long-term healthy eating habits than shedding a couple of kilos by following any of the crash diets.

Conclusion

Thank you once again for choosing this book.

You were given all the information you need about the keto vegetarian diet. Following the keto diet is quite simple. By making a few simple changes to your eating habits, you can reap all the benefits that this diet offers. The vegetarian recipes will help ensure that you stick to this diet. It is quite simple to follow the keto diet. However, changing your diet is a major lifestyle change. So, be patient with yourself and give your body a while to get accustomed to the new diet. Consistent effort, conscious eating habits, and patience are the three things you need to follow this diet. Once you do this, you will see an improvement in your overall health within no time. Also, the keto diet isn't a short-term solution. You must stick to it in the long run if you want to improve your health.

The vegetarian keto diet will certainly improve your overall health and well-being. Use the food list given in this book and make it a point to stock up on all the necessary keto-friendly ingredients. Once you have all the ingredients, it becomes easier to cook. Follow the recipes and tips given in this book to ensure that you stick to the diet. The recipes given in this book are not only easy, but will also help you cook delicious and nutritious meals. Cooking has never been this simple or easy. You no longer have to spend hours upon hours, whipping up meals in the kitchen. If you manage to do the necessary meal prep over the weekends, then cooking during the weekdays will become quite easy.

Remember that the key to your health lies in your hands. If you want to improve your health, then you must act immediately. Now, that you are armed with all the information about the keto vegetarian diet, all that is left for you to do is get started! So, get started and attain your weight loss and fitness goals!

Thank you and all the best!

References

Butler, N. (2019). Ketosis vs. Ketoacidosis: What's the Difference?. Retrieved from https://www.healthline.com/health/ketosis-vs-ketoacidosis#statistics

Comprehensive Guide To The Vegetarian Ketogenic Diet | Ruled Me. (2019). Retrieved from https://www.ruled.me/comprehensive-guide-vegetarian-ketogenic-diet/

Horton, B. (2019). What Can You Eat on a Vegetarian Keto Diet?. Retrieved from http://www.eatingwell.com/article/291617/what-can-you-eat-on-a-vegetarian-keto-diet/

Is Too Much Protein Bad for Ketosis? The Truth Behind How Much Protein You Need on Keto | Ruled Me. (2019). Retrieved from https://www.ruled.me/too-much-protein-bad-for-ketosis/

Ketone Testing - How To Test for Ketones & Ketone Test Levels. (2019). Retrieved from https://www.diabetes.co.uk/diabetes_care/testing-for-ketones.html

Ketogenic Diet Safety: Who Shouldn't Be on a Keto Diet. (2019). Retrieved from https://www.diabetes.co.uk/keto/keto-diet-safety.html

Ketogenic Diet Safety: Who Shouldn't Be on a Keto Diet. (2019). Retrieved from https://www.diabetes.co.uk/keto/keto-diet-safety.html

Ketosis and the Keto Diet. (2019). Retrieved from https://www.webmd.com/diabetes/type-1-diabetes-guide/what-is-ketosis

Mateo, A. (2019). https://www.shape.com. Retrieved from https://www.shape.com/healthy-eating/diet-tips/vegetarian-keto-diet-tips

Migala, J., & Kennedy, K. (2019). 8 of the Best Keto-Friendly Drinks. Retrieved from https://www.everydayhealth.com/ketogenic-diet/diet/best-drinks-keto-diet/

Spritzler, F. (2019). 7 Effective Tips to Get Into Ketosis. Retrieved from https://www.healthline.com/nutrition/7-tips-to-get-into-ketosis#section5

Printed in Great
Britain
by Amazon